WHOLISTIC FEMINISM

Be Happy, Be Whole! Leah Jacobson

Healing the Identity Crisis
Caused by the Women's Movement

LEAH A. JACOBSON MA, IBCLC

LUMEN
PRESS
& MEDIA

WHOLISTIC FEMINISM

Healing the Identity Crisis Caused by the Women's Movement
By Leah A. Jacobson MA, IBCLC

Nihil Obstat: Rev. Anthony Craig, S.T.L.

Imprimatur:
Very Rev. James B. Bissonette, STL, JCL
Vicar General, Diocese of Duluth

The granting of the Imprimatur is not to be understood as an endorsement of the opinions or viewpoints of the author, but rather is a declaration that the work in question is free from doctrinal error and may be published.

Published by:

Lumen Press
P.O. Box 238
Ironton, MN 56455

Produced by:

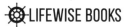

PO BOX 1072
Pinehurst, TX 77362
LifeWiseBooks.com

To contact the author: contact@theguidingstarproject.com

ISBN (Print): 978-1-7352237-0-4
ISBN (Ebook): 978-1-7352237-1-1

DEDICATION

To Josh, you are my best friend, my greatest support, and the person I want to spend every day of my life with. You have taught me what it means to be fully accepted and have opened my heart to experience the beautiful interplay of husband and wife. Because of you, I understand love. Thank you.

To Caleb, Tobias, Aliza, Ezra, Levi, Eliora, and Esther; you have taught me everything I know about motherhood. Each one of you has brought deeper understanding and love into my life, and I am so grateful for each of you. God has big plans for all of you, and I can't wait to see you live them out!

And finally, to all the great women who have come before me, with hearts for unity and sisterhood; may my work build upon all that was good and true in your work. And to all women of goodwill, that we can see the unique gifts in one another and celebrate each other.

SPECIAL ACKNOWLEDGEMENTS

To the women who helped edit and provided valuable feedback on book content: Molly Daley, Anita Morin, Anna Frient, Anna Mayer, Jamie Rathjen, Patricia Deshane, Charity Bradshaw, Stephanie Winter, Erika Pearson, and Chrissy Johnson.

To all the women I have had the pleasure to serve as a campus minister and a lactation consultant, your questions and curiosities have taught me to never stop seeking truth and knowledge.

And finally, to all those who I have worked with at Guiding Star, you all have inspired me to continue on in this work day after day. Your sisterhood and friendship and willingness to come alongside me and DREAM BIG has been a constant source of comfort for me. You are the change the world needs.

CONTENTS

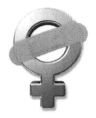

FEMALE IDENTITY

"Our physical bodies can teach us deep spiritual truths. The meaning of life, our purpose, what will bring us joy; all can be found with careful observation of and care for our bodies."

LEAH JACOBSON MA, IBCLC

SISTERS DIVIDED

Not too long ago I was mindlessly scrolling through my social media feed before bed. I came across a thread in one of the many moms' groups I belong to. It started out familiarly, "Hey friends, rough day…just looking for some solidarity. My toddler is starting to act out at daycare, and I'm not sure what to think about it. Has anyone experienced a sudden change in their kid's behavior for no reason?"

I braced myself as I looked down to the comment section, knowing what was about to be unleashed on this poor unsuspecting mother with the misbehaving tot. And so, it began.

"Why are you leaving a toddler at daycare?! Those are very formative years. You should be home with him."

"Is your child breastfeeding? If not, you should definitely start doing that again. It helps with emotional intelligence."

"Have you tried changing his diet? We cut out all food dyes, and it's done wonders for our kids."

"There is always a reason kids act out. Was he recently vaccinated? Vaccinations are suuuper dangerous."

"I think you're probably just overreacting. Kids this age act out. It's normal."

"He's obviously not well attached; you should move him back into your bed to make him more secure."

"He needs such and such essential oil...I can get you a great deal on it."

And the list went on and on. Never mind that the original poster did not directly ask for specific advice but instead was looking for solidarity and encouragement. Woman after woman responded with what they believed to be helpful direction to this mother. As with many social media interactions, the majority of the comments held a bit of criticism and strongly held opinions as to what they believed was best for this stranger's child. Most commenters were obviously attempting to self-justify or reassure themselves for their own parenting choices and didn't even attempt empathy or concern.

Many made negative assumptions about the woman's parenting style and even her adeptness as a mother. Eventually the comments devolved into a nasty argument, as they often do on social media, and the moderator jumped in to inform everyone that the comments were now disabled. The sheer familiarity of the exchange led me to ask myself out loud,

"Why are women so divided these days? Why can't we just accompany one another and be there for each other in our times of need?"

These are honest questions that point to a problem I see all around me in real life outside of social media too. There are the mommy cliques in the school PTA, the mean girl troops at the local high schools, the women at church who only invite certain women to their Bible study, and the coworkers who issue private invites to a select few to get together for a drink after work.

We are constantly evaluating other women to find the ones who are acceptable for us to commune with. It's a competition to fit in, and we're always on the hunt to find our place and our people. Most of us treat other women outside of our tribe with a degree of indifference or even standoffishness. They're just different from us. They have nothing in common with us. We don't identify with them, so why would we bother?

WOMEN'S COLLECTIVE IDENTITIES THROUGHOUT TIME

In each age of the women's movement, there have been women who have not felt at home. Over the last three hundred years, the accepted roles and identities for women in America have shifted tremendously. What has been appropriate and the ideal model of femininity in a new world was largely determined by the practical needs of the culture and environment the women found themselves in.

As America was first settled, women were needed not only as wives and mothers at the heart of the home, but they were also required to be brave pioneers settling a wild new land. They were entrepreneurs finding ways to barter their skills with one another and social architects establishing the morals of the first generations of native-born American children. Docility was not necessarily a prized trait for women who needed to negotiate and keep their families alive. Not all women thrived in this world and many surely longed for circumstances different than their own.

As the United States became organized and a governing body was established, much of the early chaos of an uncivilized world faded away, and women were expected to adapt their skills into more domestic roles, supportive of husbands and children. Survival was still a major goal at this time, and most women saw marriage and family life as the safest place to live out their lives.

The male-governed land was interested in expansion and depended upon women to stabilize their new communities and homes. Women were the backbone of our nation's growth, and everywhere women went, the towns grew and became prosperous. Most of the lives of women who lived through this time period have been lost from the historical record and forgotten. Their identities mostly unknown. Did they find joy and fulfilment in their daily tasks? Did they look back at the end of their lives and see their contributions as meaningful?

There are always notable women in every era who buck conventional expectations, and even though history is sparse in recording the lives of these tremendous women, we know they existed. We hear about women like Harriet Tubman, Amelia Earhart, Pocahontas, Abigail Adams, Annie Oakley, Katy Ferguson, Betsy Ross, Elizabeth Cady Stanton, Madam (Sarah) C. J. Walker, and many more who were notable because they simply didn't fit the norm for women at their time. Their accomplishments stood out because they were different than most other women.

Their identities were outside the collective expectations for women. They simply couldn't stay within the lines and the rules for women of their era and broke free to write their own lives. At the time, they were isolated and often ridiculed, but now they are admired because it is clear they knew their unique identities and chased the lives they knew they were created for.

Today we see millions of women struggling to find the meaning and purpose in their own lives.

Is this the life I am meant to live?

What have I done that is noteworthy?

What am I supposed to do with my life?

We value individuality and encourage our daughters to be themselves, yet so many of us are left feeling stressed out about choosing the right path and wonder about how we will leave our mark on the world.

Do career women feel more satisfied than stay-at-home mothers?

Does having wealth mean my life is a success?

Am I happy with the path I have chosen?

These are the questions we're grappling with as modern women because we can't seem to feel fully integrated, whole, and authentic in our identities as women. We're trying to do it all, and it's causing an incredible amount of stress and anxiety. We're just not finding the joy that our mothers' generation told us was available for the taking when they told us we could be anything we want to be.

We're searching for our tribes, our own little groups of friends to give our lives meaning and purpose and friendship in the everyday; while at the same time, we're guilty of judging other women's choices and distancing ourselves from them, thinking they are somehow a threat to our own identities and perceptions of success. *If she is happier than me, perhaps my life is a failure.*

> *Have we women always been so indifferent and at the same time so antagonistic toward one another?*

> *Wasn't the women's movement supposed to unite us women?*

> *Weren't we supposed to be the daughters and granddaughters of the brave feminists who fought for us to experience radical solidarity with one another?*

> *What happened to sisterhood?*

> *Is it possible that feminism itself is part of the problem and somehow to blame for women becoming so divided?*

The women's movement here in America certainly broadened the horizons for women to live out their interests in a number of different ways and smashed the societal expectation to be wives and mothers. But perhaps all these different options and ways to live our lives as modern women caused us to lose sight of what we have in common. Perhaps the "sisterhood" became too narrow in collecting just the right kind of women and was more problematic than inclusive. The sad truth is feminism has only identified some problems faced by some women and failed to give all women the tools to chart their own lives in ways that honored all of their gifts, passions, and creativity.

Maybe the rules for living a successful, meaningful, purposeful life that tell us where we belong in the modern world are wrong. Who wrote them anyhow? We are no longer trying to settle a new land and establish the laws of a new country. We don't need to fit into a neat mold for the sake of survival. We're also not trying to prove some point about the abilities of women in comparison to men; we know we're capable of so many things men can do. Why are we feeling so out of sorts with choosing our paths and defining our lives? Maybe it's time we break free from previous expectations for women and create a movement that celebrates each unique beautiful woman. I believe it's possible if we first focus on making every woman whole.

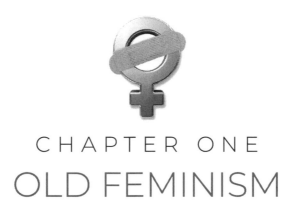

CHAPTER ONE
OLD FEMINISM

"The world will be saved by the western woman."
DALAI LAMA

Sometimes things happen in our lives that at the time are mortifying, but in hindsight you can see that this exact moment was transformational on the path you would walk moving forward. One such moment happened to me in the fall of 2008 when I was attending an evening workshop for women's studies students and the general public on the topic of women in politics.

"Don't let her tell you how to think!" the older women's studies professor screamed as she pointed her accusing finger at me. She stood in an aggressive stance, glaring at me over her wide-rimmed glasses as she leaned forward and yelled. Her graying hair was cut into a short pixie style, and she oozed authority and dominance in this setting. The classroom was her domain, and I was an unwelcome intruder.

I sat, shocked into silence in the large lecture hall at the University of Minnesota, Duluth (UMD). A hush fell over the crowd of about one hundred people as several young women quickly looked away from me and down at their feet, in obvious embarrassment of their professor's behavior toward me.

I was a young mother in my mid-twenties, with two little boys at home. I had recently left my position working full-time in campus ministry at UMD to stay home full time with my children. I was an alumna of the psychology department there, and since I still had many friends on campus who were both undergraduates and graduate students, I often found myself on campus for interesting events such as this one.

It was a way for me to get out of the house and engage my academic and political mind after exhausting days of raising toddlers at home. I was particularly drawn to the advertisements for this lecture and discussion, as the topic was women in politics and women's healthcare, and so I arranged for childcare and headed toward campus for what I hoped would be a lively dialog about women's place and influence in society.

This professor's angry outburst came during the Q and A portion of the presentation, after we had finished watching a short documentary about EMILY's List—whose motto is "We ignite change by getting pro-choice Democratic women elected to office," and another nonprofit organization on a quest to have a woman elected to the presidency of the United States by the year 2020.[1] I had raised my hand and asked the presenter, a local female politician, if she felt that Sarah Palin's recent nomination to the Republican ticket as the vice-presidential candidate was a sign of women moving closer toward the goal of becoming president. The elected official answered carefully with typical politician speak and said that while she could appreciate the accomplishments of Mrs. Palin politically, she would not personally be supporting her as a candidate.

Since she hadn't really addressed my question, I pressed on further and asked if this nomination should be seen as a sign of hope for young women who may want to aspire to political careers but that also want families like Mrs. Palin. I shared that I was a young mother preparing to go back to graduate school for a career in women's health and that I felt encouraged to see a mother with young children so vocally calling for women to embrace their motherhood alongside their careers.

It seemed a hopeful sign to me that motherhood would not necessarily cement my exit from academic, professional, or political life. I also shared that I appreciated Mrs. Palin's positions with regards to women's healthcare issues as they more closely aligned to my own, but that I felt women often were not able to talk about shifting the terms and definitions of women's rights in this day and age.

I saw several young women nod and smile at me and could feel that the freshman women's studies class required to attend the workshop was on my side. They too could appreciate seeing a strong, opinionated woman being put on the presidential ticket and didn't understand why other women would refuse to support her. I mean, wasn't feminism about women uniting to help propel all women forward together?

It was at this moment that the professor jumped to her feet and began her angry tirade against me. She screamed that any woman who would not support unrestricted access to "women's healthcare," such as Sarah Palin, was not really a feminist but rather a pawn for the powerful men behind her. She scolded her students and reminded them that their duty as women's studies students was to fight for and protect "women's rights" against anyone who would challenge them—me included.

She erroneously assumed that I was a political plant in support of the Republican party, and therefore, I should not have a voice about women's healthcare or feminism. She looked at me with so much hatred and contempt that I wanted to crawl under my chair! I was caught completely off guard. Her tone and accusations had shaken me to my core, and I was so embarrassed.

FRACTURED FEMINISM

As unfortunate as this experience was, it served as a landmark on my journey into women's healthcare and feminism. This was the first time I personally experienced such a brazen and obvious attack against my opinions and my dignity, signaling my exclusion from a group of women I had previously hoped could be my sister activists.

Prior to this encounter, I believed there was room at the table for me in the modern feminist movement. I honestly believed the movement would value the diverse opinions and intellectual contributions of uniquely positioned and qualified women to speak to their own experiences of being women in this day and age.

As I stood in front of that lecture hall over a decade ago, I only felt hurt and confused by this professor's anger toward me. However, as the shock wore off and I asked myself what her motivations could have possibly been to attack me, a fire was fueled within me to understand the history and future projection of feminism. Who was this movement benefiting if my voice and opinions didn't belong?

That professor couldn't have been more wrong about me when she assumed I was there to push Republican politics. She didn't know I truly was very interested and invested in the field of women's healthcare, and I wanted to call myself a feminist alongside her. She had no idea I attended local mother's support groups that leaned very liberally to the left, or that I was a recipient and a strong supporter of government programs to help women and their children.

I was not a pawn of the Republican party and had actually voted most recently for a pro-life Democrat in our district. I was never given the opportunity to refute her angry assertions and libel because she had figuratively slammed the door in my face. The possibility of building a future relationship with me was killed by her close-mindedness. She assigned me to some other team and made it clear I was as good as an enemy to her.

To this day, I can't quite get over the irony of this older female professor, telling a class of young impressionable women to not listen to the opinion of another woman because it contradicted her own. "Don't let her tell you what to think; let *me* tell you what to think" is basically what she said.

This wasn't what I believed feminism to be about. Her abuse of power in this situation mimicked everything I had been taught to question as someone who considered herself a budding feminist. It made me pause to gain my bearings on the movement I thought I was a part of.

As their professor, this woman held a position of authority over these students, and her public shaming of me made it clear to them that they had better not question or think for themselves under her watch. The aggressive domination of these younger women reeked of the unequal power distribution that had previously existed in some areas of American society. It looked and felt exactly like the male domination or "patriarchy" that feminists claimed to fight.

It had zero feminine qualities such as hospitality and relationality that I would have expected to see in a movement led by women. I had naively thought feminists would appreciate and welcome strong-minded and opinionated women to the movement and nurture younger women to stand up and speak, even if the opinion differed from their own.

This event was bewildering and began what would become a small obsession for me. I had to understand how and why women became so divided against one another, and why feminism felt more like thought-control than women's empowerment. I left that night having realized two things:

1. I didn't understand the goals of feminism.
2. I obviously did not belong in the modern feminist movement.

I would come to learn that I was certainly not alone. I initially wanted to be a feminist because I thought it was about advocating for all women. I still believe this is what feminism can be, but it starts with acknowledging where it went so wrong.

WHAT DOES IT MEAN TO BE A FEMINIST?

I'm not going to lie; feminism is one of those things I've gone back and forth on a number of times. I've never been entirely sure that feminist was a title I wanted to take up or identify with. Certain aspects of the movement seemed attractive, like fighting for equal dignity and equal pay for equal work. However, just as I was about to sign up to attend a march or buy a button, I'd run into something so opposed to my logic and reasoning I'd have to opt out of feminism. Even though there are aspects that I have supported, the movement as claimed by that women's studies professor just doesn't mesh fully with who I believe myself to be, and it doesn't really seem to be addressing the issues that I care about most as a woman. And I don't think I'm alone here either.

When polled, just 20 percent of Americans—including 23 percent of women and 16 percent of men—consider themselves feminists. Another 8 percent consider themselves anti-feminists, while 63 percent said they are neither. But asked if they believe that "men and women should be social, political, and economic equals," 82 percent of the

survey respondents said they did, and just 9 percent said they did not.
[2] Although Americans may support and identify with the purported
purpose of feminism, they still don't seem to want the title. Perhaps this
can be chalked up to the confusion about what the title means? I know
I was confused.

What does *feminism* actually mean? According to the Merriam-Webster
Online Dictionary, the word *feminism* was the most searched word in
their internet database in 2017; it was even chosen as their Word of the
Year.[3] It experienced a 70 percent spike in searches from the previous
year as millions of people around the world tried to make sense of what
the century-old movement means for modern times.

Merriam Webster's Dictionary defines feminism as:

1. the theory of the political, economic, and social equality of
   the sexes
2. organized activity on behalf of women's rights and interests[4]

This seems like a straightforward and simple word on the surface, yet it
holds baggage and ties to social movements that make it hard to fully
understand. Although we may agree and identify with some ideas we
associate with feminism, many of us disagree with issues that seem to
be nonnegotiable for other feminists. We may believe that women are
equal to men, but does that mean we must also support all the other
ideas that seem to go along with the word *feminist*?

UNDERSTANDING THE FEMINIST MOVEMENT

If we're going to be talking about the women's movement and the role
of feminism in the current issue of female identity loss, it's important
to have a basic understanding of it and its goals throughout the last two
centuries. I certainly didn't understand what exactly feminism was and

wasn't when I was a teenager, so I want to do you a solid favor and give you an overview before we really jump in.

The women's movement (the term *feminism* wasn't widely embraced until the 1960s) has been at work in the United States for about two hundred years, with a more recognizably organized movement just over 125 years old. In most college women's studies programs, it's taught that there have been three major waves of feminist activity and that we are now beginning a fourth wave.

The first wave of feminism began in the second half of the 1800s and centered on the main issues of suffrage, slavery, and abolitionism. It ended with the ratification of the 19th Amendment in 1920 that granted voting rights to all women. The second wave of feminism got its feet under it as a social movement in the 1950s and shifted its gaze toward upsetting social expectations for women to be homemakers and mothers. It helped launch the sexual revolution of the late 1960s and 1970s and then morphed into a third wave of activism in the early 1980s.

This third wave of feminism was less directed at issues pertaining only to women but at a broader spectrum of issues relating to gender generically and toward gaining that elusive status of "equality." I would classify this wave as more ideological and theoretical than the previous two waves because it philosophized more on the possibilities for a non-gender-conforming society than it did on advocating for the rights of women.

This puts us currently at the beginning of what will historically be recalled as the fourth wave of feminism. Some say it is already well underway with the rise of something called "intersectional feminism" and "nonbinary feminism," but I think the possibilities for this next wave of activism are endless and that there is still plenty of room for wholistic feminists like me (and hopefully you) to have an influence on the women's movement.

Understanding the waves of feminism is a necessary framework for you to start out with. Each wave has key issues that it promotes, and at times, they directly conflict with the work and views of previous feminists. The next thirty years will tell us if fourth-wave feminism has succeeded in creating a better society and culture for all women. We'll know we've progressed when we see women claim their unique individual identities and create a culture that truly makes room for differing viewpoints and experiences.

VICTIMHOOD

It's important to understand that there is no defined "feminist charter" or rules that are enforced by some group at the top. It has mostly been an organically grown grassroots movement, made up of very diverse individuals, each bringing their own ideas to the conversation. Certain issues come forward as key for the movement to address, but until groups like the League of Women Voters and the National Organization for Women were established, it was merely a common sentiment of victimhood that united and propelled the women's movement forward.

When I think back to the experience that I had with that professor over a decade ago, I can now see more clearly that what we were experiencing was an identity clash. We were two very different women who both were attempting to take up the same title of feminist, which meant different things to each of us. I was in the naivete and can concede that the feminist movement I was claiming membership in really didn't even exist in the mainstream yet.

The feminism I was describing was in its infancy and had no well-known leaders or documents to define it. It also had several ideological differences from her version of feminism, which was far more mainstream and accepted. I didn't realize it at the time, but she likely counted me as anti-feminist because I did not subscribe to a victim mentality. In every wave of feminism previously, women had united as victims of at least one of the following oppressors (real or imagined): men, our bodies, or Mother Nature herself.

THE FIRST WAVE:
VICTIMS OF A MALE-DOMINATED SYSTEM

In the first wave of feminism, women united as victims of unjust laws created by men and broken relationships with men. They gathered together at the Seneca Falls Convention in 1848 and laid out their grievances with their treatment at the hands of an all-male system. They published the Declaration of Sentiments, which listed sixteen accusations against men, fifteen of them starting with the words "He has" and then continuing with the charge against men for the position of women in society. They did not waste words on outlining the unique gifts of women and how their contributions to society were priceless; they simply borrowed from the Declaration of Independence and stated their equality. They began their new declaration by altering the text of our famous founding document to highlight the injustices against women.

> *When, in the course of human events, it becomes necessary for one portion of the family of man to assume among the people of the earth a position different from that which they have hitherto occupied, but one to which the laws of nature and of nature's God entitle them, a decent respect to the opinions of mankind requires that they should declare the causes that impel them to such a course.*

We hold these truths to be self-evident; that all men and women are created equal; that they are endowed by their Creator with certain inalienable rights; that among these are life, liberty, and the pursuit of happiness; that to secure these rights governments are instituted, deriving their just powers from the consent of the governed. Whenever any form of Government becomes destructive of these ends, it is the right of those who suffer from it to refuse allegiance to it, and to insist upon the institution of a new government, laying its foundation on such principles, and organizing its powers in such form as to them shall seem most likely to affect their safety and happiness.[5]

These small changes, such as adding the word *woman*, may not seem monumental to us now, but at the time the notion that women be granted equal voice in governance and law was unheard of. The original women's movement in the United States began from a common starting point—we women are all victims of men and the system they have established. At this point in time, most women met the social obligations of marriage and motherhood resulting in little diversity in the female experience, creating a strong collective identity as wives and mothers. The Declaration of Sentiments had the ability to speak on behalf of women collectively because most women did conform to the strict societal expectations set forth for their behavior.

Motherhood and raising children were realities experienced by most women, and so they used their united voices to make changes that brought greater respect and improved the situation for women. The solutions they championed, such as rights to property, inheritances, and custody of their children, represented the needs of all women, and the movement generally succeeded in uniting the majority of women.

There was unspoken unity about the experience of being a woman, and very few women were exceptions to the norm.

Although there were some women who chose not to be involved with the suffrage movement and some did actively oppose suffrage, very few women thought laws giving wives and mothers rights to their children and property were a bad thing. The identities of wife and mother unified the movement toward combating the injustice of women's treatment by men.

SECOND WAVE: VICTIMS IN OUR HOMES AND TO OUR BODIES

In second-wave feminism, something very different happened. The victim status that would unite this movement was not universally accepted and was championed by a privileged group of women who did not understand the goals and hopes of most women. A few social thought leaders, such as Betty Friedan and Gloria Steinem, stepped forward with books and magazine articles claiming to represent the experience of all women, portraying women as struggling and isolated housewives who were captives in their own homes. These leaders stated that women were once again victims of an unjust system, yet they struggled to articulate the problem. As Betty Friedan said, the problem really had no name.[6]

There was indeed a sense of unrest in many women in the post-WWII era as the country readjusted to peacetime with men back at home. But instead of taking the time to really understand that the issue had to do with women not finding fulfillment and joy in their roles as wives and mothers, they surmised that these roles themselves were the problem. They rallied against the expectations of previous generations about becoming wives and mothers and declared all women were oppressed by the collective identity of housewife.

However, this victim identity did not resonate with all women, and second-wave feminism floundered from the beginning to find unifying principles and a collective identity that women related to. Many women were content as wives and mothers and found it confusing that they were being called to rise up and join this new movement.

In the excitement of launching this new social revolution, second-wave feminism failed to uphold wife and mother as noble options for women and failed to advocate for changes in policies in the workplace and all places outside the home. Without changes to the existing workplace infrastructure, being fertile and having babies became the barrier to adopting the new identity of the career woman that was being pushed on young women.

Marriage became the enemy to education as colleges had no expectation to accommodate married student couples and had no leniency for pregnant and parenting students. Motherhood became a liability for women wanting to climb the career ladder as workplaces certainly were not going to provide maternity leave or flexible options for women to thrive as both employees and moms. It wasn't really being a housewife that was making the women of the post-WWII era so restless; it was a world that told them motherhood and the home required a woman's full attention and that they were not capable of doing anything beyond that.

There was literally no way for her to succeed as both wife and mother and career woman without massive changes to the system. Sadly, these changes were not the main concern of second-wave feminism.

THE SEXUAL REVOLUTION

The timing of the sexual revolution played a major role in shifting the problem from being housewives, to blaming the female body and its fertility for holding women back. Had the sexual revolution not come into full swing at exactly this moment, the second wave may have kept its focus on the issue of women's discontent in the home and been able to champion solutions that allowed them to maintain the identity of wife and mother and find creative work outside the home.

However, with the growing movement claiming sexual expression as a source of fulfillment, it became an obvious solution to encourage women to reject the roles of wives and mothers completely and to suppress the biological consequences of recreational sex, also known as "free love." Suppressing women's bodies and fighting for abortion rights made sense if you could convince women that being a career girl having sex with as many people as you wished would bring you fulfillment.

Young women were now encouraged to sacrifice their identities as successful wives and mothers to be successful, sexually expressive career women. Books like Helen Gurley's *Sex and the Single Girl* made the argument that female fertility and marriage was an easy trade-off for fun and fulfillment.[7] It was a trade that millions of women eagerly made, and one that they and their children and families have paid the price for.

The "problem that had no name" began by acknowledging women's restlessness in the home, and gave the solution of creative work outside the home, but without the systems in place to support and respect women as wives and mothers in their desire to be both in and out of the home, fertility and children became the barrier to women finding the fulfillment that was promised.

The one thing that should have united all women as something more than victims ended up being the very thing they began to fight against—***our female bodies and the biological reality of our fertility***. Ironically, the truest and purest point of authentic unity and understanding between women; our female bodies and womanhood, became the common enemy that ultimately united the second-wave feminists.

THIRD WAVE:
VICTIMS OF MOTHER NATURE

In third-wave feminism, the enemy was articulated as the stereotypical expectations that follow gender and the question of whether gender identity is an issue of the mind or body. In this wave, victimhood status was granted to anyone who experienced mistreatment or discrimination because of their natural bodies and the societal expectations placed on them. This included men and people from all backgrounds, especially minority groups.

Because the sexual revolution was just wrapping up at the start of this wave, and the two movements were so closely intertwined, third-wave feminism focused especially on redefining societal standards for sexual activity and sexual attraction. In a carryover from the previous two waves of feminism, men and women were not necessarily viewed as complementary counterparts. The binary male/female relationship was no longer assumed to be the ideal. The body and its natural sex organs were an inconsequential aspect of human fulfillment and were seen as a possible barrier to finding one's truest self. The mind and the body could be separated, and the women's movement ballooned in numbers as the issues surrounding gender identity and expression were now limitless.

Any person whose mind tells them something different than what their body displays is now a victim of Mother Nature's cruel joke. And the sad irony of this is that many of the people who experience this difficult internal divide are pushed to make this dissection of mind from body by the rigidity of our lingering shallow societal standards for male/female behavior. Just as the second-wave feminists fought for ways for women to express themselves outside the tight confines of wife and mother in the home, third-wave feminists now fight for new words and expressions that would allow us to be ourselves outside the overly simplified guidelines that are provided for male and female behavior.

But by accepting the lie that the mind and body can be separated from one another, we do not get at the issue of the limitations of shallow gender stereotyping. Instead, we only cause greater confusion and chaos by saying we are victims of nature, which leaves women even less sure of what will ultimately bring them joy.

FROM VICTIMS OF MEN, TO VICTIMS OF OUR BODIES, TO VICTIMS OF MOTHER NATURE

The shifting identities of feminism have led us to a place where men, our bodies, and our very female nature are now seen as barriers to our fulfillment and happiness. We've been led to believe that we can't trust the things that we find ourselves naturally drawn toward and are told that that equality comes when we are free of obligations for relationships, free of the burden of caring for dependents, and free of the rules of nature.

Sisters, this is insane. We know it in our hearts. We want to believe that we're not victims, but we don't know who we are because we are throwing out all the guideposts to finding the best versions of ourselves. If we can't trust men, our bodies, or even Mother Nature, what are we supposed to trust? Are we supposed to just close off the rest of the world and look only at ourselves to find our purpose? It may sound good, but that's not how it works. We are not islands, and we do not find ourselves in isolation. Our gifts, passions, and purpose are evident only when we are creating and giving it away, to others. We are made for relationship. We can only find our whole selves when we consider and make peace with our relationships with men, our bodies, and Mother Nature.

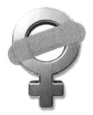

CHAPTER TWO

OUR TRUE PRIVILEGE

"We can no longer ignore that voice within women that says: 'I want something more than my husband, and my children, and my home.'"
BETTY FRIEDAN

I grew up in a place mostly untouched by the rhetoric of second- and third-wave feminism. I lived on a small dairy farm in central Minnesota, in an agrarian community where the Future Farmers of America (FFA) was a big deal and 4-H clubs were the height of my social circle. Every day I saw strong women all around me, using their uniquely feminine minds and bodies to work alongside their husbands and earn a living as farmers and housewives.

Through the humdrum of daily life, the farm wives at church, my aunts, and my own mother taught me about womanhood. They taught me the beauty of a woman's mind, body, and spirit in such a beautiful and natural way. Feminist rhetoric did not seem to apply to us because the obvious differences between the sexes were accounted for on a daily basis and Mother Nature was in charge.

In the world I grew up in, right at the transition of second- to third-wave feminism, the ideologies and gender theories of feminist scholars took a back seat to the practicalities of everyday life. In rural life, gender stereotypes bend with more fluidity because of the work that must be done. Husbands and wives operate as partners on the farm, and the breakdown of all the work that must be done does not fit neatly into boxes marked "man" or "woman."

Women baled hay and milked cows alongside men, and I grew up with the same expectations to do chores in the barn along with my older brother. My older sister chose to mostly stay in the house and do the dishes each night after supper, while I rushed out to the barn to avoid housework, but even she couldn't escape picking rocks from the fields on hot summer days.

Farm life doesn't respect traditional gender roles when there is work to be done; any able body has to help out. So, while feminists were fighting for the right for women to work outside the home and do everything men can do, the women doing the hard and dirty jobs on the farm would have loved to experience the comforts that were common to their city sisters. Nature and responsibility had a much stronger pull on women than so-called women's rights and entitlements to do this unsavory work.

None of the neighbor farm ladies that I can recall spent much time or money on clothes, makeup, or beauty products. My mom and aunts were about as low maintenance as women come. It would have been considered an incredible luxury for the women of my childhood to have had their hair and nails done. Farm wives simply didn't do that; they couldn't do that between feeding cows in the mornings, getting kids off to school, cleaning the house, ordering seeds and farm supplies, paying the bills, grocery shopping and making meals, sitting on the tractor all afternoon, and feeding and milking cows before bed at night.

The gender-fluid goals of the second and third wave of feminism were not what farm wives were hoping and fighting for; they were the reality for women living a life with little luxury or privilege. Farm wives were not "free to express masculine traits" and do "men's work"; it was simply expected of them.

OCCUPATION: HOUSEWIFE

One of the most influential voices of the second wave of modern feminism came in 1963. She was an obscure, middle-aged woman, mother of three children, who published a book that launched a societal revolution. This woman was smart; she was college educated and received several scholarships and academic awards.

She had worked as a journalist and political activist, but at the time that her momentous book was published, she was working from home as a freelance writer. She was politically active much of her life and just a decade earlier worked at a popular magazine. But because modern antidiscrimination laws were not in place, she was let go due to her second pregnancy. Her famous book was a social commentary compiling the stories of many women of the time and concluded that society had narrowed the acceptable sphere for women to exist only as housewives, thus causing women great personal distress and loss of identity. This woman was Betty Friedan and her book was *The Feminine Mystique*.

It is no exaggeration to say that Friedan's book was groundbreaking and changed the course of many women's lives. It was a sensation when it was published as women bought copies to share with their friends and sisters. The year it was released it became the best-selling nonfiction book and sold 1.4 million copies.[1] To date, it has sold over three million copies. Her book breathed life and gave a united voice to second-wave feminism in the second half of the twentieth century.

The key assertion in Friedan's book was that women were limited in their career options and that many were pressured into becoming housewives, not understanding its constricting nature. Friedan said that this restriction of women's talents and creativity in the role of a housewife was resulting in women feeling desperate and depressed as homemakers. She called this condition of widespread discontent "the problem that has no name."[2] The cure she proposed to this malaise was for women to find creative work outside the home.

> "It is urgent to understand how the very condition of being a housewife can create a sense of emptiness, non-existence, nothingness in women. For women of ability in America today, I am convinced there is something about the housewife state that is dangerous."[3]

Years following *The Feminine Mystique,* women flocked into the workforce and now, fifty-seven years later, most women participate in paid labor outside of the home. In 2019, there were 76,852,000 women age sixteen and over in the labor force, representing close to half (47.0 percent) of the total labor force.[4] Women held 51.8 percent of all management, professional, and related occupations.[5]

THE PRIVILEGED FEMINIST

Betty Friedan insinuated in her second-wave feminist manifesto, *The Feminine Mystique,* that there was a greater purpose to women's lives beyond their family and home. This statement comes from the incredibly privileged perspective of post-WWII American prosperity and security. Friedan herself lived in a large home and had hired help with her children, luxuries for any woman past or present.[6] The subtle undertones of victimhood that painted the beautiful gifts of a loving husband, children, and a home as oppressive show the obvious privilege that this wave of activism was born of and brings into focus the separation from reality that those who promote this worldview live under.

Betty Friedan was free from the burdens of necessary work outside the home, although this freedom to be at home was exactly what felt like a prison to her. She perceived her creativity and individuality were stifled by societal expectations to be a homemaker.

Post WWII was a time when strong gender roles were enacted and societal pressure kept the majority of women in the home and away from many creative outlets. The relative ease and comfort of this lifestyle could not be fully appreciated by Friedan and many other women. Her first-world affluence brings into focus her naivete of difficult living conditions around the world and frames her discontent as a luxury that many modern women can't afford.

For women who have lived through the recent recession and economic instability, and who must work to keep their crushing debt from burying them alive, the idea of staying home with their children, with no pressure to financially contribute, is a daydream. Many modern women longingly search images online of homemaking ideas during their lunch hours at work. They get up early to pack their young children off to daycare and at the end of the day scramble to make supper, do homework, and tuck kids in before falling into bed themselves, exhausted.

Ironically, it is in places of privilege we see feminism most actively engaged in rooting out supposed inequalities. You very seldom see women's marches and rallies where women are most in need. Feminists do not march on behalf of the more than 200 million girls and women alive today who have been cut in thirty countries in Africa, the Middle

East, and Asia because of female genital mutilation. Their true needs, such as clean drinking water and improved medical care, are a mystery to most modern feminists.

This idea was summarized in Obianuju Ekeocha's "Open Letter to Melinda Gates." This Nigerian women's right's activist is one of the most powerful modern-day feminists:

> *"Please Melinda, listen to the heart-felt cry of an African woman and mercifully channel your funds to pay for what we REALLY need."*[7]

Gates pledged to infuse 69 of the poorest countries in the world (most of which are in sub-Saharan Africa) with $5 billion in family planning initiative to curb population and increase access to contraception. Ekeocha's plea for Gates to see the effects of this funding on the lives of African women went unheard as she predicted, "[Gate's pledge will]" ensure that the African woman is less fertile, less encumbered, and, yes, she says, more "liberated." With her incredible wealth, she wants to replace the legacy of an African woman (which is her child) with the legacy of "child-free sex."

Perhaps this is why the women I grew up with had a hard time identifying with those in positions of leadership in the feminist movement. The concerns of feminism just didn't resonate with our real-life needs I saw around me.

THE AMERICAN DREAM

A few years ago, I took a "check your privilege" test on a website that no longer exists and was surprised to learn that, according to that site[8], I was considered below average for privilege in America. I guess I shouldn't have been surprised because I am part of the first generation to receive a four-year college degree in my family. My parents' income was always very modest, to exaggerate greatly, and we would have been eligible for every form of government assistance available, although, on principle, they would have never accepted it. I grew up in a rural, economically depressed area with little access to culture or outside influence.

As a young child, my family experienced housing instability and even ended up living in my uncle's workshop for several months. We were building a barn and making the old farmhouse on the farm my parents purchased livable (it didn't have running water, doors, insulation, or even interior walls), so technically we were homeless during that time. I remember wearing my snowsuit indoors to stay warm those first few months as we moved into that old house. I don't recall having new clothes very often as I wore hand-me-downs from my older sister, which she got from my older cousins and aunts.

According to the privilege-checking website, all these things put me on the underprivileged side of things, even though I'm racially privileged as a white person. But I honestly never truly felt poor or disadvantaged growing up because I always knew there were people out there who had it much worse. Yes, I knew that money was tight and that the pea green snowsuit I inherited from my older male cousin wasn't exactly cute. I was acutely aware that the budget eyeglasses I was forced to wear made me look a little like that kid Ralphie from *The Christmas Story* movie, and that most of the kids in my class could afford a new lunch box each year, but I didn't spend time worrying about those things. It was just the way it was, and I was healthy and happy.

I grew up in a time and place when having a husband, children, and a nice home were still the American dream. I never felt like a victim of my poverty or my female body because no one in my early life ever made me feel that way. Our female bodies were sometimes less able to do the really hard physical things that the men could do on the farm, but we were also very special because we were able to carry new life and nurture babies. Pregnant women were treated special.

I always understood that some people were alone in this world and that I was blessed because I had my family and we were all happy and healthy. We were not privileged enough to complain about the good things in our life. Success meant a happy and healthy family and time to be together. The life that Betty Friedan pushed back against and second-wave feminism rejected was, and I believe still is, the dream of America's underprivileged.

The goals of third-wave feminism, of gender sameness, and interchangeable sexes are nonsensical to many average Americans. I believe that most women who live close to Mother Nature reject the feminist narrative because it does not adequately account for biological realities, nor does it honor the beauty of our natural bodies and see the purpose for the male/female difference.

STRESSED OUT

The stresses that modern women are feeling are palpable. Whether you're a single woman just heading off to college, a working mom trying to make a life for your family, or a successful career woman at the top of the corporate ladder, the feelings of "not doing enough" or fearing that you're "doing it all wrong" persist. The discontent and second-guessing didn't go away when our career and relationship options opened up.

Since the 1950s, women have gone to college in record numbers. In 2015–2016, 56 percent of college students were female, and 44 percent were male.[9] From 1990 until 2015, the number of males enrolled in college increased by 41 percent, while the number of female students rose by 53 percent.[10] We've outpaced men in obtaining higher educations, and we've also shifted the average marrying age of women to a decade older, with the median age at first marriage reaching its highest point on record in 2018: thirty years old for men and twenty-eight years for women, according to the US Census Bureau.[11]

We have used those single years to climb the ranks of the corporate and political ladders and have managed to close the gender pay gap a few cents, well at least arguably for younger women anyhow.[12] But what have all these achievements and successes cost us? These numbers mean little when women are not experiencing feelings of happiness and integration in their work and personal lives. Instead of looking like the images portrayed on the cover of *Cosmo* magazine depicting successful single gals living sexually exciting and happy lives, we seem to be experiencing an identity crisis of epic proportions, not sure at all anymore of what we want.

In an October 2017 article by Ada Calhoun called, "The New Midlife Crisis," Calhoun reports that women who are approaching midlife are experiencing symptoms of depression, anxiety, and identity confusion at an astonishing rate. Nearly 60 percent of Gen Xers describe themselves as stressed out. [13] A 2009 analysis of General Social Survey data showed that women's happiness "declined both absolutely and relative to men" from the early '70s to the mid-2000s. [14]

Our mental health has suffered tremendously in the past two decades. A more recent analysis done by *The New York Times* in 2018 found that "white women over [age] 45 account for about one-fifth of the adult population but account for 41 percent of antidepressant users, up from about 30 percent in 2000. Older white women account for 58 percent of those on antidepressants long term."[15]

What in the world is going on?! Why are women floundering so badly at a time when our career and relationship options have opened up and many of us are pursuing the creative outlets outside the home that

Friedan predicted would bring us joy? Calhoun points to the instability of many of our childhoods, overwhelming education and home debt, failed relationships, parenting concerns, and unfavorable economic conditions as key reasons that many women my age and older are feeling tremendously stressed out.

We've tried to prove we can do it all on our own, and it's making us miserable. More importantly, Calhoun also pointed to the discriminatory workplace practices that are often lobbed at women who are experiencing the hormonal shift of perimenopause and menopause. Many women are dealing with the confusing symptoms of the grand climacteric event of their life while also fighting to step into leadership roles in the workplace and guide their growing children out of the home and into college.

These women are wearing a dozen different hats, and each one of them is all-consuming. And they're not even allowed the time or space to talk about or acknowledge the incredible physical transformation they are experiencing because it's not polite conversation. Ladies, we've done this to ourselves by accepting a fragmented and masculine framework for professional behavior that separates all of our identities into neat little boxes that are only opened one at a time and in appropriate situations. We've maimed our right to be whole, which is what we truly need to live fully integrated lives, and we've obviously gotten something about female fulfillment wrong. Perhaps we've failed to truly understand our identities as women?

WOMAN: WHOLE AND UNDIVIDED

What if instead of telling our daughters what success looks like, we let them show us what female creativity, and connectedness, and authenticity look like?

Woman, the mature female figure, is powerfully creative. She looks like strength, is clothed in dignity, with her head held high in awareness and knowledge of her goodness. Don't we all want our girls to grow up to be like her?! Woman is essential to the balance and health of society with her uniquely female mind, body, and spirit.

Our world is hurting because we do not see and value the sacred feminine within each of us and within each other. We have the power to create space for our girls by carving out and claiming the collective voice that is our birthright. It starts by truly seeking unity with our sisters and throwing out the victim mindset just because we are women.

We are good and we were created exactly as we were supposed to be. There is nothing wrong with our female minds, bodies, or spirits, and while there are differences in experiences and opinions among women, we have more things in common with one another than different. We can't keep focusing on our differences if we want to create a women's movement that will make each woman whole.

FOURTH WAVE:
VICTIMS OF CHAOS

The first Women's March on Washington in January 2017 highlighted a rise in what has been called "intersectional feminism." The term is nearly thirty years old, but it seems to be reaching its heyday right now as several different types of feminists attempt to find common ground with one another to revive and unite the fractured feminist movement.

Intersectional feminism was termed by American civil rights advocate and scholar of critical race theory, Kimberlé Williams Crenshaw in 1989. Crenshaw believed feminism must take into account additional outside identifiers for each woman beyond her femaleness (such as race, ethnicity, social status, sexuality, and religion) when searching for solutions to the problems facing women because these can contribute to increased oppression.[16] So, for instance, a black woman who identifies as a lesbian could experience further levels of oppression than a straight white woman, which would theoretically make it more difficult for her to receive equal status with other humans.

This type of feminism is currently very attractive for many who want to find common ground and grow a large united social justice movement capable of addressing a myriad of injustices all at once. And for the time being, intersectionality seems to be giving some much-needed energy to the feminist movement. We are seeing people from various civil rights and social justice causes line up alongside feminism in the name of intersectionality. The Women's March in 2017 included diverse sponsors such as Black Lives Matters, Planned Parenthood, Occupy Wallstreet, PFLAG (Parents and Friends of Lesbians and Gays), and Natural Resources Defense Council (just to name a few).[17] These groups give an indication of the broad range of causes that united under the banner of a "women's march." One reporter noted prior to the march: "The Women's March has drawn plenty of detractors who question what such an event can accomplish, especially given the diverse messages of the many environmental, civil rights, labor and women's groups that are sponsors and partners." [18]

Some of these organizations did not even have women as the primary recipients of their services, but their energy and support went a long way in bringing people together to march for something. While the energy of having so many allied groups in attendance caught the attention of the world, this is not a viable long-term solution to the internal problems challenging modern feminism. The woman is losing her collective identity completely under a feminism that focuses more on political allegiances than women's bodies.

FEMINISM, SIMPLIFIED

There are problems at the very core identity of feminism that if not addressed will result in the movement for women becoming simply the movement for human equality. We must look back to the core identity of feminist activism and see if there is still something strong enough to direct this movement forward in a unified way. Victimhood will only push us further down a pathway of identity loss and confusion. We must understand and promote what is good about being women and make that the heart of our movement.

Interestingly, Merriam-Webster dictionary noted that the definition of feminism has been altered many times over the history of the word in their book.[19] It first appeared in their print edition as early as 1841. Its original definition was simply "the qualities of females." That's it. No political agenda or movement associated with the term in the very beginning.

Perhaps there is wisdom in the simplicity of the very first definition of feminism, and this simplicity is something we need to reflect upon and be careful to preserve moving forward. If we continue down the path of intersectional feminism and nonbinary feminism, it's possible "women" will eventually be erased from the "women's movement." If we're not careful and we do not keep our female bodies and our common female experiences central to our advocacy, it is entirely possible that our authentic needs as females could be brushed aside by our other identifying characteristics.

When the additional outlying human identifiers of oppression become the core of feminism, it is women who will be hurt and excluded the most. As one philosopher once stated, "Feminism without femininity is a sham."[20] How do we ensure fourth-wave feminism will be about and for the benefit of all women?

At the March for Women, we saw that despite hundreds of thousands of women coming together to express their beliefs about the dignity and equality of women, many women still felt slighted and left out because they did not agree with some organizers and sponsors about what is good and healthy for women. Many men felt more welcome at the Women's March than some women.

The event was laced with stories about sponsor organizations being removed from the list and women boycotting the march because they held political opinions deemed opposing to some undefined charter of feminist principles.[21] It would appear that the movement for women ironically divided women and this time went as far as telling women who think differently that they do not belong in the feminist movement. (That was certainly a deja vu moment for me as I thought back to being screamed at by that feminist professor.)

Bringing in so many diverse political causes created an atmosphere where women felt divided politically and stripped the feminist movement once again of its purported goal to unite and advocate on behalf of all women.

At this critical point, when feminism is trying to find and assert its true identity, we must look again at the original definition of feminism and ask two simple questions:

1. What are the unique qualities of only females?
2. Does our DNA, our female biology, have anything to do with the experience of womanhood?

The answers to these questions must remain at the center of every organizer and leader's mind in the women's movement. If we move away from the commonality of womanhood and instead focus on human rights in general, we may, in the end, actually cause feminism to lose its female identity and fail women instead of strengthening the movement.

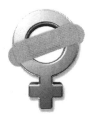

CHAPTER THREE

OUR RIGHT TO KNOW OUR BODIES: FERTILITY, CHILDBEARING, BREASTFEEDING

"I think it's the worst thing that we do to each other as women, not share the truth about our bodies and how they work and how they don't work."

MICHELLE OBAMA

My husband, Josh, and I spent the first three years of our marriage living in the campus ministry Newman House on the edge of the UMD campus, surrounded by student housing and roughly 10,000 college students. We were young and right out of college ourselves, enthusiastic about starting our married life together.

We opened up our home to the students in our ministry, and before long, our first home together became the home-away-from-home for dozens of college students. There were young people in and out of our house at all hours. Most of the time, I loved it because the cozy environment allowed for intimate conversations with students about the big issues they were currently dealing with. Oftentimes, someone would knock on my office door and ask if we could talk "for just a few minutes," which usually meant I should put on the tea kettle and settle in to hear about their recent breakup or help them try to figure out what to do with their lives.

About four months into our young marriage, we found ourselves unexpectedly expecting our first baby. It wasn't something we were trying to achieve, nor explicitly avoid, but the swiftness of our fertility caught us a bit off guard as we realized we would be parents before our twenty-third birthdays. Between pregnancy naps on the couch and making weekly meals for around seventy-five students in my tiny kitchen, I was answering students' questions about relationships, marriage, sex, fertility, pregnancy, childbirth, breastfeeding, and being a new parent.

Many students had never been around a young married couple with a new baby so they had all sorts of questions about what this phase of life was like. As one of the only pregnant and parenting mothers on the campus, I found myself the de facto expert on these issues, not because I knew that much, but because these students knew even less.

I was going through my own massive transformation from young woman to young mother as my body seemed to take over and do things I had no ability to direct. It was a learning experience of complete trust and surrender only possible through experiencing my body's own abilities and strengths.

My previous notions of "feminine power" and "feminine abilities" slowly gave way to a new way of looking at myself and other females in our society. I watched in awe as I grew a human life, then birthed, then nourished it outside myself with nothing other than my breasts. Where I used to see the supreme proof of our abilities as matching and outpacing men, I can now see an innate beauty within women that has nothing to do with emulating masculine traits.

I can see the uniqueness of our bodies and minds and have grown to treasure the presence of these attributes in our world. I now recognize our fertility, our childbearing abilities, and our fitness to provide breast milk to our children as absolute beauty and gifts to society. These acts give dignity to another being by virtue of our attention and care for them.

As a young mother, I learned the importance of mothering, not only for my baby, but also those around me who needed my attention and care. We tell our children they matter by mothering them. The same is true for all the people in our lives. The mothering instincts and selfless love women bring to society, both as physical mothers and spiritual mothers, are gifts to all humanity, not just their own biological children. These things set women uniquely apart from men and elevate us to a status deserving of reverence and recognition within our society.

We are capable of things man can, at best, mimic but could never replicate or replace perfectly. Our strength is in our natural feminine essence. Our acceptance and elevation of these feminine traits is important for the health of society. My body taught me deep spiritual truths about purpose and meaning like nothing else had before. What I found was that the world needs more mothers, but I didn't know this until I became a mother myself.

As someone who has become passionate about teaching other women about the beauty of their bodies and the amazing things they are capable of doing, I have become increasingly troubled by the negative perceptions of many women toward their own natural "feminine abilities."

Early on in my conversations with many of the young women on campus, I noted there was often a fundamental difference in our beliefs about our roles, bodies, careers, and motherhood. The conversation might start out innocently with a student asking me about how I was feeling and if I was nervous to give birth, and then it would evolve into a discussion about how she was not planning to have children for several more years because her parents expected her to pay off her student loans before she started a family. Or she would carefully ask when I was planning to wean my one-year-old because in her opinion that just seemed really old for a baby to still be nursing. I occasionally even got questions about whether or not we were going to continue using natural fertility awareness methods of family planning when we announced that we were having a second child.

These questions led to countless discussions about:

- societal expectations for women
- how sexual relationships affect women disproportionately in our culture
- the benefits of breastfeeding
- natural fertility awareness methods for relationships and women's health
- ultimately, what these young women desired to do with their lives

Many hours were spent telling them their natural bodies and their natural desires for relationship were created beautifully and they were not the problem. I explained the basics of fertility tracking, the natural cycle of hormones each month, and assured them that these were vital parts of their female identities.

I'd listen as they would talk about how their boyfriends would never let them go off the pill, or how they didn't think they were smart enough to chart their fertility. I repeated the lines over and over again to countless students: "Your body is NOT the problem! You CAN live a fulfilling life. You are smart and capable. You are NOT a mistake."

WHY WEREN'T WE TAUGHT THESE THINGS?!

As grown women, we need to come to terms with the miseducation many of us received in our younger years about our gifts and our natural body's abilities. Most of us were never taught that we are only fertile for approximately 100 hours per cycle, when sperm life and cervical mucus are considered.[1] Heck, we were probably never even told that we need cervical mucus to get pregnant, or that it has noticeable changes throughout the month, signaling increasing and decreasing fertility. Most of us didn't realize how quickly our fertility would decline after age thirty-five, and we certainly didn't know that for every year on the pill it's estimated that our cervical crypts, which make that magical cervical mucus, age two years.[2]

Of course, we are upset about the lack of information provided to us by previous generations. They didn't give us the tools to understand our own bodies or how to integrate their natural functions into meaningful and fulfilling lives.

Realistically, they probably didn't know to question the ideas the feminist movement or the medical community were selling them. Most lacked the knowledge or courage to think any differently because information about how their own bodies worked was not readily available to them. Most likely they were not the ones promoting the falsehood that our female bodies were a problem but rather were the passive participants in a shifting worldview.

It does no good to villainize previous women's activists if we're trying to move forward in a united way. We must forgive their ignorance and commit to avoiding the circumstances that led them to take such erroneous positions against women's best interests. What young women want is the information to make life decisions informed by their biological reality. We all deserved to have this information.

LOSS OF GENERATIONAL GUIDANCE

I was eleven years old when I had my first period. Fifth grade. I think I may have been the first girl in my class, but I'm not really sure since this was not something we generally talked to each other about. Thankfully it happened while I was at home. And luckily, earlier that very same day we had the presentation on puberty from the school nurse and were given some pads and pamphlets explaining what to expect. Less than twelve hours after being gifted that "first period kit" at school, I put it to use.

My mom had to sign a permission slip for me to attend that class, which led to us having a conversation about my changing body. I was lucky my mom talked with me about this, as it seemed most of my friends' moms didn't. My mom had more knowledge of the menstrual cycle and cycles of fertility from growing up on a farm. She shared the basics of fertility with me in broad terms and explained that it simply meant I could get pregnant once I started my period.

As awkward as it was for me to sit through, I appreciated my mother sharing with me her own story of NOT being told what to expect with the onset of monthly menses. She laughed and cringed as she shared her embarrassing story of being eleven years old and waking one morning to the blood in her underwear. She had no idea if she had somehow hurt herself, or if she was dying! She had not been told anything about her cycle of fertility and was completely convinced that something was gravely wrong with her body.

She was too afraid to tell my grandmother or her two older sisters, and instead set off on the half-mile walk to school like normal that morning. By mid-morning, my grandma called the country schoolhouse and asked the teacher to send her home. She had been doing laundry and making beds and found the hidden evidence declaring her third daughter's first menstrual cycle.

My mom ran home as fast as she could, afraid that my grandma would be upset with her about the mess, and also terrified to tell her that she was bleeding to death! When she arrived home her mother handed her a menstrual belt, a huge awkward pad, and a small booklet explaining menstruation. She told her to go to the bathroom and read the booklet. No reassuring words of "It's all right!" or "You're going to be okay" or "Don't be afraid, you're NOT dying," just instructions to go into the bathroom and read the booklet.

When she read it, things made much more sense as she recalled her two older sisters' strange secrecy over the past year. All three sisters began cycling within a year of one another, yet it still came as a complete surprise for my poor mom. At some point, my grandmother briskly explained that this is something that will now happen every month, they had products to help her manage it, and to talk to her sisters if she had any other questions. She thought, *Relief! I'm not dying!* Followed by dread. *Every month! But why?*

We do not have rites of passage for our girls built into American culture. There are no menarche celebration ceremonies and often not even words for girls to tell their mothers what is happening to them. A girl will whisper quietly that "it" has started and the following shushed conversation with their mother cements into her young impressionable mind that this is not something to be celebrated. Our daughters are not transitioned into understanding the change of their status from child to young woman. Nor are our boys experiencing the rites of passage that signal they are now young men with life-giving powers. This is tragic and is contributing to a prolonged childish approach to fertility. Understanding the basics of our female bodies has not been something the women's movement has put much time or energy into. As much as it has shouted rhetoric like, "My body, my choice," it has dealt with our bodies largely as an inconvenience and focused more on defining successful and fulfilled lives outside of our natural and healthy reality.

THE FEMININE ABILITIES

After the numerous conversations I had with young women while in campus ministry, I was inspired to go back to grad school to get a master's degree in Women's Health and Wellness. I had come to terms with my own knowledge gaps and decided I wanted to work in women's healthcare. I am now an International Board-Certified Lactation Consultant (IBCLC), and every day I am able to teach women that they are not victims of their bodies, but rather they have the ability to change the world for the better through them. My work is an amazing gift to me because I get to see women go from a place of doubt and distrust to empowerment and confidence in themselves.

While writing my final master's thesis, I really challenged myself to look at the state of women's health, including the mind, body, and spirit connection. I could tell so many women felt disconnected. Their bodies weren't feeding their spirits, and their minds seemed to be at war with everything the body was trying to do.

I thought a lot about what it means to provide healthcare services to women and how I could speak truth about the goodness of their whole being. I worked to create a picture of what an integrated women's health system should look like in treating women as whole unique beings. During this research period of my life, I coined a phrase to explain the unique functions of women's bodies; I called them the "feminine abilities," for lack of a better term.

The main realization I came to was that women's bodies performed three biological functions completely separate from the basic functions that both male and female bodies can do. These distinctly feminine abilities are **ovulation, gestation,** and **lactation.** They really are like superhuman powers when rightly viewed.

I looked around at how culture was speaking to young women about these tremendous abilities and found the messages were mixed, confusing, and sometimes completely inaccurate. It became much easier for me to understand why so many college-aged women were distrustful of their bodies and why women in general were slow to embrace their fertility, childbearing, and breastfeeding abilities.

We've allowed our culture to blame our bodies for all the inequalities we experience as women. In every woman's magazine, there are multiple articles that communicate our worth in terms of our sexual appeal, our careers, and our freedom from long-term commitments such as marriage and children. The single, sexually available woman is portrayed as the height of happiness and success. The only mention of our feminine abilities is in ads for ovulation-suppressing drugs, information on delaying pregnancy, and virtually nothing about our breasts lactating, except a million tips on maximizing breast cleavage with the WonderBra and makeup tricks.

Rather than elevating culture to appreciate and support women's bodies, we settled for a culture that says our bodies are for sexual pleasure only, making the right to alter, suppress, and destroy our fertile, life-giving female bodies the supreme "women's right."

SEX ED AND HEALTH CLASS

Indoctrination on the problem of the female body starts young. As you probably know, it is pretty standard in the United States for public, and many private, schools to teach sex education classes starting around fourth to fifth grade—that's roughly nine to ten years old. These classes are usually an hour or two long and are taught by the school nurse or some other health educator. They explain some of the basics of puberty, and for girls, a "starter kit" and quick lesson on menstruation.

Unfortunately, most little girls (and boys) leave these classes unable to explain what the onset of the menstrual cycle and puberty really means to them biologically. Many do not understand that they will now be able to take part in the greatest of human endeavors, reproduction. Most girls simply retain the idea that menstruation is embarrassing and shameful.

As these children grow into teenagers, they will take part in more health classes offered by the schools and sometimes churches. The focus will shift to the consequences of using their bodies in the ways they are naturally begging to be used. This next set of classes (usually called "Healthy Choices" or something similar) is focused on one of two things:

- suppressing fertility
- suppressing all sexual activity to avoid unwanted pregnancies and sexually transmitted infections/diseases

These health classes instill fear in young people about the risks and consequences of sexual behavior and leave them with the idea that natural sex is "unsafe." Condoms and contraception are pushed, but nowhere in these early educational experiences are young people taught to recognize the shifting hormones women experience each month. Nowhere are they encouraged to fully understand the process of ovulation and how to track female fertility. Nowhere are young men told that fertility is a shared act and that they are always fertile; therefore, they should be aware of their responsibility in engaging young women for sex.

We owe it to younger women to instill in them a sense of respect and care for their fertility. By learning about their bodies at a young age, they will begin a relationship with their bodies that's built on trust, and they will want to protect this precious part of themselves. We can also teach them to recognize the type of men who are capable of valuing and cooperating with a natural female body free of suppression.

NEW AND UPDATED AWARENESS

Our girls have spent hours learning how to hide their periods and what pills to take to trick their bodies into not getting pregnant, and yet they do not know the most basic signs of a natural cycle of fertility. Things like changing cervical mucus, the temperature increase after ovulation, and breast tenderness are all things that avoid our detection because we simply were not taught to pay attention to them.

There are many methods of natural family planning that have rates of efficacy rivalling artificial contraceptive methods, but sadly these advances have been overlooked because society has settled for a method that suppresses feminine fertility instead of honoring and working with it. Many people discount fertility awareness methods by ignorantly dismissing them as the "rhythm method."

Most are unaware of medical advances that have brought us incredibly accurate sympto-thermal monitoring, cervical mucus monitoring methods, lactation amenorrheal, and sympto-hormonal monitoring that is now possible in the comfort of your home. Charting cycles is also a vital indicator of our overall health as women, and we have been wrongly deprived of this basic knowledge for more than a generation.

It is now very possible for women to pinpoint their hours of fertility with certainty and be able to make family planning decisions with the same levels of accuracy of most artificial family planning methods. To learn more about these medically relevant methods of family planning, visit FactsAboutFertility.org.

Now, imagine the confusion and frustration that will take place twenty years later when some of these sub-educated girls, now women, are dealing with infertility. Fertility was pushed aside, suppressed, and ignored, and now the thing that was avoided and feared for decades has escaped. What's even more sad is many women today have never heard about the medical advances of natural methods of fertility care, such as the Creighton NaPro Technology Model, which is three times more effective at achieving a pregnancy than in-vitro fertilization (IVF). [3]

With more than 6.7 million women in the United States struggling with infertility currently, IVF will only help 0.44 percent (or 28,200) of these women annually.[4] The reality is, IVF falls tremendously short as a solution for infertility because it does not seek to identify or treat the causes of infertility; instead, it attempts to bypass them. If the problem is a hormonal imbalance, endometriosis, cysts, or a number of other issues, IVF does nothing to correct these problems. It takes a healthy and hormonally balanced body to get pregnant and sustain a pregnancy. Many women just need help getting things in order first, not a total removal of the process from their system. Sometimes it seems that our desire to control all the outcomes gets in the way of respecting the process.

PREGNANCY, LABOR, AND DELIVERY

My husband and I have been tremendously blessed with good fertility. Having worked with many women who struggle to conceive children, it is not something I take for granted. If you are someone who has experienced the trial of infertility, I want you to know that I see you and share a sense of frustration at how unfair this world can be. You are good, and your body still deserves tremendous respect and care. I am rooting for you to be able to live out your motherhood in the way you are uniquely called to.

I have given birth to seven children, and medically speaking, each experience was very different.

- Three of them were induced.
- I had epidurals for four of them.
- Three were totally unmedicated.
- Two were born in the water.
- Six were born in three different hospitals.
- One was born at home.
- Four were delivered by obstetricians.
- Two were delivered by family practice doctors.
- One was born with the help of a certified professional midwife.

Each labor also varied with one lasting thirty-three hours and another lasting about forty-five minutes. I have learned so much about myself through giving birth. Sharing about each birth can be likened to the war stories many veterans tell years after the battle. The details remain vivid and etched in—the scars and traumas as well. None of my births were especially complicated, yet some recoveries took much longer. With at least two of them, I dealt with postpartum mood issues.

At the time I felt very isolated and alone, but when I look around me now, I can see I was certainly not an anomaly. It's estimated that as many as 9 percent of women deal with much more severe post-traumatic stress disorder from their childbirth experience.[5] How we approach pregnancy and birth and our expectations can have an impact on how we feel about the experience afterward.

I took birth preparation classes at least four times, not because I couldn't remember what was said, but because I wanted to see how the different settings presented the information. I found that depending on the provider and the birth setting, the worldview on birth was very different.

Example One:

In the hospital that hosted the region's only level-3 NICU, birth was presented as an inherently dangerous medical process that would often require the support of pain medications and interventions to safely be accomplished. The class here gave us a lot of information about medications we could request and warned that only the father of the baby was welcome to enter the labor ward.

No outside birth support, like doulas, would be allowed. We were also discouraged from writing up birthing plans because we were warned that they often led to disappointment. They also had a policy of only delivery in the lithotomy position (on your back with your feet up in the stirrups), as this was a teaching hospital and they thought this was the easiest way for new providers and students to learn. Never mind how this might negatively affect the mother and baby.[6]

Example Two:

In stark comparison, for my second baby, I attended the natural childbirth classes hosted by a naturopathic doctor and midwife. These classes were completely different in tone and focused on mind management and relaxation techniques to lean into the coming "waves" of contracting uterine muscles. Pain was not something to fear, and we were told over and over again that our bodies were meant to do this.

This class took the time to explain each stage of labor both biologically and emotionally and equipped mothers to not fear the process. We were told to labor and deliver our babies in whatever position our body wanted to be in and watched videos of women birthing while pulling on ropes in squatting positions, giving birth in water, and even using birthing seats. It was a completely different approach, and it stuck with me because I knew that I was being told the truth about my body. The women in these videos looked so connected to themselves and the process and the outcomes showed that letting their bodies lead led to better outcomes.

The tendency of modern medicine to "take over" is an incredibly masculine approach, to control and manipulate the birth process, supposedly for the ease and convenience of the laboring mother. The rise of women using terms such as "birth rape" to describe their childbirth experience indicates that some women feel dominated and forced into submission in the birth room. Aggressive interventions may come from a place of concern for both mother and child, but at what cost to women's well-being?

Giving birth is one of the most vulnerable, sacred experiences of a woman's life; for her to feel trauma instead of joy afterward shows that we have failed to understand women's needs in childbirth. For women who understand how to surrender and how to trust in the design of their bodies, pregnancy and childbirth can be incredibly spiritual and an empowering experience.

FEMINISM AND NATURAL BIRTH

> "Birth is not only about making babies. Birth is about making mothers—strong, competent, capable mothers who trust themselves and know their inner strength."
>
> BARBARA KATZ ROTHMAN

The women's movement hasn't really known what to do about having babies, and throughout the years, feminists have taken drastically different stances on it. While early feminists advocated for highly medicated births as a right, some later feminists claimed that birth choice with regard to medical practices was a critical element of bodily autonomy. Author Barbara Harper talks about the defiant attitude toward medical convention that developed in the second wave of the women's movement in her book *Gentle Birth Choices*:

> The women's movement in the 1960s and 1970s created an atmosphere that led women to question medical practices concerning their bodies. The feminist

movement spent much more time claiming the right to abortion than it did in claiming the right to natural childbirth; burning bras was not necessarily an effort to make breast-feeding easier.[7]

The zeitgeist of a female revolution was a defiance of previous norms and pushing new frontiers. Unfortunately, the issue of natural childbirth was brushed aside, as it no longer fit the feminist narrative of a childfree lifestyle. But only fifty years earlier, birthing practices were the issue that women were discussing. Where and how to give birth was a topic of much cultural debate and disagreement among women as birth moved from the home into hospitals.

CONTROLLED BIRTH

A huge shift away from home birth rose sharply at the turn of the twentieth century. "While 95% of American births took place at home in 1900, only 50% did so in 1939."[8] Our first US president to be born in a hospital, James Earl "Jimmy" Carter, was born on October 1, 1924. His birth came right in the middle of the tidal wave of women choosing to birth in modern hospitals. [9]

While much can be said about what was lost in terms of sisterhood when birth was no longer attended at home by women, we need to consider the effects on our identities as we moved into a male-regulated hospital system. What followed the surge of women into the hospitals was the development of strict protocols and procedures to standardize the practices of birth. All of these practices were meant to make birth safer, quicker, and less painful, but some may have resulted in robbing women of the experience altogether and left them wondering about their own abilities to naturally birth their children.

As childbirth moved from the home into the hospital setting, women lost many of the comforting and relaxing measures they had in the security and familiarity of their homes surrounded by sisters and friends. As a result, many women experienced great anxiety and pain in childbirth in the hospital setting. Because of this, the demand for pain relief increased and even led to the formation of a society to advocate for extreme forms of pain management, including "twilight sleep."[10]

Some women began to demand as much medication as they could get their hands on, championing it as a "women's rights" issue. There was little to no research on the safety or long-term effects of all this medication on women and their babies, and so for nearly fifty years, the art of natural childbirth was lost in a flurry of public opinion and rhetoric pushed out by the popular medium of women's magazines.

The "twilight sleep" era of the 1910s–1960s is probably the most notable embarrassment to American medical birth history both for its lack of sound medical evidence-based outcomes, and also for the way it often degraded women in a precious moment that should result in great empowerment and joy. Instead of joyful accomplishment and relief, many women experienced only a dull, floating sensation.

The combination of the drugs morphine and scopolamine caused women to fall into a state where "they could still feel and respond to contractions but supposedly would not remember what happened. [...] In addition women had to be carefully guarded from hurting themselves, which sometimes required them to be strapped or tied to the bed for hours as a result of the hallucinogenic side effects of the drug."[11] Today the pictures and stories of these births seem tragically unnecessary with the knowledge we now have, but this was the norm at the time.

In the 1960s and 1970s, there was a backlash against how medicalized hospital birth had become. A new wave of midwives began to rise up in the midst of the sexual revolution and called for birth to be moved out of the hospital setting. Perhaps the most famous of these midwives was Ina May Gaskin and her birth community, affectionately called The Farm.

The women who flocked to The Farm to give birth were largely considered "hippies" or social extremists, but the ideology they embraced was that women were not broken and that they did not need to be "rescued" from giving birth. They presented a new model of care for expectant mothers and for their deliveries. They began questioning how we give birth in America, and their questions are still resonating today.

Despite spirited arguments within the medical community, there has been a rise in women who are opting to move out of the hospital setting for home births. Home births increased by 77 percent from 2004 to 2017, whereas birth center births more than doubled.[12] Some are attributing the rise in home births to Ricki Lake's documentary *The Business of Being Born* and the many recent books by midwives and doulas outlining the supposed dangers of hospital births as opposed to home births. Although the women's movement is not actively promoting the benefits of natural childbirth, there is almost a stronger ally for natural birth from celebrities in Hollywood and online who are beginning to express childbirth as a rite of passage they want to take part in.

BREASTFEEDING

"When we trust the makers of baby formula more than we do our own ability to nourish our babies, we lose a chance to claim an aspect of our power as women. It is an act of female power, and I think of it as feminism in its purest form."

CHRISTINE NORTHRUP

Since becoming certified as an IBCLC in 2012, I have practiced in both the hospital labor and delivery department and in my own private practice, home-based setting. As a mother to seven breastfed children (I've breastfed for roughly a decade of my life), I can tell you a lot about the practicalities of breastfeeding and how this natural feminine ability shapes us in ways we had no idea were possible.

Breastfeeding is biologically the last of the natural feminine abilities that we come to, (ovulation, gestation, then lactation) and often our understanding of our fertility and our childbirth experiences can taint our expectations for breastfeeding. When we have a new baby in our arms, whose needs demand we figure out our final feminine ability of lactation in a very short span of time, any doubt about our bodies' abilities come rushing forward.

The vulnerability of postpartum hormones, the pain that can follow a difficult delivery, plus the sleeplessness of caring for a newborn set the stage for new mothers to feel a wide range of emotions, many of which are negative and self-defeating. New mothers need seasoned mothers around them to nurture and guide them into this new role. Breastfeeding a baby is the final biological maturation of our fertile female bodies, but it is the beginning for most of us to understand the symbiotic nature of ourselves. Caring for a new baby leaves us fully surrendered to the experience of being a woman.

While it may be hard to believe now, breastfeeding has not always been embraced by those advocating for women's health. If we study the history of the women's movement and how it has interacted with the delivery of women's healthcare, we can see each wave of feminism has recognized and advocated for acceptance or rejection of the natural feminine abilities to different degrees. But in the current culture of "breast is best," it's hard for many to believe that women's rights activists could ever have had a problem with women's right to breastfeed.

In 1971, an all-time low national breastfeeding initiation rate of only 24.7 percent was hit.[13] Less than one hundred years before the low was hit, nearly 100 percent of babies were breastfed in the immediate postpartum period. Prior to the drop of breastfeeding rates, which began in the late 1800s, nearly all American women breastfed their babies. "In this era before access to ice and refrigeration, breastfeeding was especially important during hot weather. Therefore, mothers never weaned during the summer and customarily breastfed their babies through at least two summers."[14]

This practice began to change near the end of the nineteenth century as infant milk-replacement formulas were developed, and many mothers began introducing cow's milk into their newborn's diets in order to wean them by three months of age. During the height of the second wave of feminism, only one in four women even attempted to breastfeed their newborns. Why? This shift was due to a number of reasons, but societal messaging to women about their abilities and expectations around their priorities were likely of great influence.

My own mother was told in the late 70s that "only poor women" breastfed their babies and was asked if she needed help to purchase formula. Luckily, she didn't listen to anyone and breastfed all of her children, even after cesarean sections, which most women were told at that time made breastfeeding impossible for them. When I was weaned from the breast, I went straight to raw, organic cow's milk fresh from the bulk tank in our own milk house.

Even though we were poor, growing up on a dairy farm had its advantages. Feeding babies raw cow's milk was another thing that only poor women did at the time, and I'm sure some felt sorry for me that I didn't have the "benefits" of formula as a baby. (For some of you who may go to tremendous lengths now to find raw, organic cow's milk, you can likely appreciate the irony that I, the daughter of a poor farmer, was given this instead of formula. How times change.)

Thanks to groups like mother-led, Le Leche League International, and aggressive educational promotion by our government's public health division and the CDC, breastfeeding rates have been slowly rising since the 1970s to the present-day initiation rate of approximately 83 percent. [15] There is still some disparity in breastfeeding initiation rates between cultural and geographical demographics in the United States with fewer non-Hispanic black infants (68.0 percent) ever being breastfed compared with non-Hispanic white infants (85.7 percent). However, the current rate of infants ever being breastfed in the US has met and exceeded the goals of the Healthy People 2020 Project of 81.9 percent by the year 2020. [16]

The fact that this mark was met two years early is a tremendous testament to the multiple organizations and government programs working together. It should give us hope that public perception and practices for women's health can shift dramatically in the span of a generation when we work together for a common good.

FEMINISM AND THE FEMININE ABILITIES

Betty Friedan spoke often about the unequal burden placed on women to care for the children and how it was women who suffered the most when couples started a family. Friedan, and many other feminist leaders, discouraged breastfeeding as a way to find independence.

Author Jen Bracken-Hull wrote,

Breastfeeding in America in Friedan's generation was the exception. Until even recently, breastfeeding women were completely excluded from public venues. In order to participate in regular public activities, women had to give up breastfeeding altogether. Additionally, during the 1970s many feminists expressed an antipathy toward reproductive functions, viewing children as restrictions on women's accomplishments. Over the centuries, they observed, women had been reduced to a set of biological functions, contributing to society primarily through the birthing and nurturing of children.[17]

There are still some feminist academics who are so wrapped up in an ideological vision of what the "equality of the sexes" means, that they neglect to acknowledge the reality of our natural bodies and what has been proven time and time again to be in the best interest of the health of humanity. There remains a belief in many feminist circles that being fertile, having babies, and breastfeeding will impose constraints on women's success and lessen their opportunities for recognition outside of their maternal achievements. I look to women like suffragist Elizabeth Cady Stanton, the mother of seven, and Supreme Court Justice Amy Coney Barrett, also the mother of seven, and I smile. There's hope for me, and every other mother out there.

Third-wave feminists, like author Joan B. Wolf, say that breastfeeding should be opposed by feminists because it perpetuates patterns of unequal responsibility in parenting. In her 2010 book, *Is Breast Best?* Wolf, a professor of gender studies, questions the scientific research about the benefits of breastfeeding. Despite hundreds of studies that point to measures of health beyond just the nutritional advantages for the baby, Wolf avoids addressing the important issues of maternal health and bonding and simply states that benefits to mothers and babies are "exaggerated." [18]

She insists that fathers can serve as a substitute for mothers and essentially states that men and women are interchangeable as parents, thus contributing to gender inequality on issues relating to motherhood. She warns against a cult of "total motherhood" in which women are encouraged to find purpose in their role as mothers, because in her view, what they are doing can also be done by men and therefore has little value. And here she is entirely wrong.

MOTHERS MATTER

The gender similarity/interchangeability framework many feminist scholars are advocating is at the core of third wave of feminist theory, and it should be alarming to anyone who wants to improve the conditions in our society to benefit women. This worldview is the greatest threat to achieving authentic gender equality for women because it refuses to recognize that women's bodies are doing something completely unique and tremendously valuable. By refusing to acknowledge biological differences and the benefits of women's biological contributions to society, we will continue to create laws and policies benefiting the male-normative culture we live in.

We value things both men and women can do more than the unique things only women can. This is dangerous and downplays the value of our female bodies. Modern feminism has been obsessed with making it possible for women to achieve the same opportunities for success that men have, but it has completely ignored that we are capable of things men could never even hope to achieve with our reproductive abilities. We should be proud of our creative capacity as mothers.

Our feminine abilities will be a strike against women as long as we allow a male-normative culture to set the bar for success. By insisting that breastfeeding has no benefit to children, Wolf and other third-wave feminists play into the idea that what we do as mothers can be replaced by bottles and that our unique contribution as breastfeeding mothers is basically worthless to our children and society. We are only "successful" when we acquiesce to models of male domination over nature. This assessment is limiting and flawed, and we as women can lead the way in defining what success is for mothers and all women, without asking men to tell us that it is valuable.

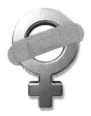

CHAPTER FOUR

THE MALE-
NORMED WORLD

"Instead of ignoring our differences,
we need to accept and transcend them."
SHERYL SANDBERG

Working as a lactation consultant affords me an intimate front-row seat to the challenges of new motherhood and the bond between mother and baby. It is a sacred space, and I am honored to be welcomed in to assist as new mothers navigate the changes to their bodies postpartum. I field dozens of questions about the mechanics of lactation and the hormone shifts of a new mother's physical body; but sadly, one of the most common lines of questions I run into in my private practice is how to navigate going back to work. New mothers wonder if they'll be able to continue breastfeeding when they return to the workforce, which usually occurs around six weeks after giving birth. The anxiety in their questions is palpable, and they seek more affirmation from me as they get closer to the day when they know they will leave their baby with someone else and go back to work full-time.

Their bodies, not nearly fully recovered from their recent pregnancy and delivery, are finally getting into the rhythm of the "fourth trimester" with a semi-established milk supply and a happy baby, and they know they are about to jeopardize the dynamic, possibly irreparably. I do what I can to teach them about pumping and remind them of their legal rights to take pumping breaks at work (unpaid of course)[1]. They do their best to store up as much milk in the freezer, and we talk about realistic expectations and goals for how long they will be able to continue nursing.

For many mothers, their breastfeeding journey will end shortly after returning to work, as the closeness and frequency required to maintain a long-term nursing relationship with their baby is no longer possible. Our lactating breasts simply don't understand or care when our fifteen-minute pumping breaks are scheduled, and they often won't cooperate and let down their milk to a cold, mechanical pump. Our bodies crave our babies.

Sometimes I note a sense of relief in mothers' voices as they talk about life "getting back to normal" with going back to work, but more often I see mothers struggling to justify why they need to leave their baby at this young age. Oftentimes, it's for reasons like staying current on their resume, or how they don't think they could handle being home all the time, as if working full-time or being home full-time are the only two options available. Many women legitimately need to work to pay off school loans or to make ends meet in their home. They are conflicted, yet the drive for success in the workplace or the pressure they feel to provide for their families often win out, and they check off another box on their endless list of things that women must do in order to be considered successful. Working mom, check.

A MAN'S WORLD

Many women will find when they return to the workplace as a mother, that it no longer is as accommodating to them as it was when they were childless. Second-wave feminism did not understand the ramifications of painting motherhood and our biological abilities as oppressive. They could not understand that by normalizing the alteration of women's biology there would be no need to create laws and policies to serve women who opted to live fully in their female bodies and embrace their procreative abilities.

By ignoring the physical realities of being women, mothers were pushed into a workforce that had no idea about the needs of women's bodies. Men held no responsibility for the challenges that women would face in this new world because these had become "women's issues," and most women were content with the solutions of altering, suppressing, and destroying the natural abilities of women's fertile bodies. Society and the workforce were not going to change to accommodate women's bodies; women's bodies could change if they wanted a seat at this table.

Feminism's solutions to women's discontent in the home grew upon the false assumption that men were not going to put women's rights first and, therefore, removed them completely from their solutions for equality. Women were not going to wait around to receive a solution from men. Women alone held the reigns for creating equality, and they grasped at the right to live the lives their husbands were living.

One of the greatest ironies of the strategies employed by second-wave feminists to create equality is that instead of creating a new norm in society that allowed women to flourish outside the home, they further entrenched a "male-normative" culture as the mark for success, which left many women floundering to adjust their natural gifts and talents in order to succeed. Women today are the recipients of a cultural expectation to carry on and get back to work within weeks of birthing a new human being. It's ridiculous, but we either play this game or sit out altogether. And it doesn't get any easier as we age; in fact, for most women the pressure increases as the demands for our time and attention in our lives increase. Men know little about the multiple arenas the average woman balances in any given day. A work day is no exception.

THE SYSTEM IS RIGGED

The second wave of feminism declared equality would come from women sharing an equal place in universities, the corporate world, and having financial freedom from men. Friedan's goal to liberate women from lives of boredom and drudgery in the home has been largely met in the last half of the twentieth century. Women are now free to pursue any career path they want, and there are no opportunities closed to the modern American woman. We experience a level of freedom and opportunity never known to women!

Feminism promised us that this freedom would provide true happiness. However, if we look around, we clearly do not see the type of freedom and creative expression our grandmother's generation was seeking. Can we definitely say that women are now better off? Are women happier now than before the push for career and sexual freedom became the mark of a successful life?

By most accounts, modern women are definitely not happier than women who first embraced career over family life.

> Every year since 1972, the General Social Survey has asked a representative sample of American adults how happy they are. In 1972, women reported being a bit happier than men. Each year since, despite the achievements of feminism, women's reported happiness

has declined, both in absolute terms and when compared with men's. Around 1990, the sexes passed each other, and since then, women have reported being less happy than men, and less happy than their mothers and grandmothers were at the same stage of life.[2]

Now, nearly six decades after the second wave of the women's movement sold a worldview of how women could feel empowered and happy, many modern women are simply feeling burned out. We are tired of spending our days feeling pulled in a million directions. Those of us who are mothers often feel guilty for everything we do, or don't do. If we work, we fear we're damaging our children by our absence. If we stay home, we worry we're becoming a "helicopter parent." If we're single, we feel undue pressure to work twice as hard as men in the office to succeed in the workforce.

There is simply no way to do it "right" in a world that has set up an impossible expectation for women to do it all. We feel the weight of expectations to be college educated, to establish a career, while finding the perfect spouse and becoming financially secure. We're supposed to have it all together before finally having perfect children that live in our beautiful house in a nice neighborhood. Ironically, we end up back in a comfortable house with a beautiful family as the end goal, but we've added in a bunch of prerequisites before it's deemed acceptable to live the life Betty Friedan encouraged us to escape.

Second-wave feminism failed us as fertile female beings when instead of creating a world where women's unique gifts and contributions could be appreciated both at home and in the workplace, the movement unwittingly degraded some of the things that bring us the most joy and purpose in life. By holding up the workforce as a superior sphere for women to be in, the women who chose to stay home began to be seen as "less than" women who chose to go to work—less sophisticated, less educated, less creative, and less motivated, although that usually was not the case. The women that I grew up watching were incredibly hardworking, innovative, and smart, yet they would have been viewed as uneducated and underachieving by the feminists of their day.

FAILING WOMEN

Instead of society making room for and accepting all women completely as we are, wherever we are, with our female minds and bodies intact, second-wave feminists allowed and even advocated for us to change ourselves physically to fit into a man's world outside the home. We insisted on the right as women to change ourselves, and yet the feminist movement failed to make the outside world more female friendly, thus perpetuating the idea that being female is at the core of the problem.

We told women to go to work but didn't demand for work to accommodate the desires of women to live lives of purpose and meaning as mothers. We didn't even ask to be acknowledged as unique from men, with our own sets of strengths that could benefit employers. Instead, we insisted we could do and be everything a male employee was. It would be many years before things like the Strengthsfinder assessment highlighted women's unique contributions, such as empathy and positivity, and acknowledged how helpful these attributes are in creating a healthy workplace environment.[3]

We betrayed our uniquely female minds and bodies and said we could effortlessly become infertile and unattached to others who might need us. We even allowed the practice of artificially stripping the female body of its truly creative capacity to become mothers through daily contraceptive use to become commonplace. We unwittingly adopted a worldview that saw our fertile bodies and feminine minds as part of the problem.

When Friedan painted the workplace as a place to liberate women from the boredom and monotony of the home, she adopted a male-normative culture with its markers for success and happiness. This meant that the game women were playing to earn the accolades and awards that signified success were all set up years in advance and favored the type of player that was single-minded, without distraction, and ruthless in pursuit of the goal. In other words, men.

The things women naturally excel at and enjoy (relationships in particular) were not counted as valuable contributions. Many women moved from the home with its self-paced lifestyle and time for conversations with our children and friends, and occasional volunteer activities, into demanding work days full of deadlines and quotas.

What if we could check out of this current system and reimagine a new one? A new system that doesn't require us to alter, suppress, and destroy our natural feminine gifts and bodily autonomy to be successful? Could we create a new type of feminism capable of bringing women true happiness and unity? I'm certain we can, but it starts with the expectation that women will be allowed to flourish fully as themselves.

UNHEALTHY COMPETITION

A woman's body performs *natural* and *innate* functions. For example, every little girl will eventually ovulate. Every little girl will eventually have the capacity to breastfeed. This is natural. Science and medicine have little to do with these abilities in most cases. Here's the problem. When society teaches women to suppress and distrust their bodies, it is also teaching women to suppress and distrust nature.

A deep trust in the reality of nature and natural order fosters a positive relationship with one's female body. When we can accept that the way that we were made as female is truly good and not in any way lacking, we can explore and find the type of life that will make us feel integrated and whole. We cannot run from our nature as women. Nor should we ignore the nature of males or feel inferior because of our biological differences.

Modern society celebrates male-normative standards for health, productivity, and success. This is confusing because accepting these standards interrupts the natural female biological reality. In order for us to perform like men, we need to push a lot harder in some areas and totally neglect others. It's hard to win as a woman when winning means being male. Society has elevated so many things that come easily to men and require no major alteration of their bodies or minds. For example, climbing single-mindedly to the highest levels of the corporate ladder, competing aggressively in physical and athletic feats that require extreme strength, and having the liberty to move about unattached to others are not easily achieved for a healthy, normal woman.

Society is not set up to accommodate women's natural bodily functions and her innate relational bonds to others. Access to childcare and maternity leave is not always easy to obtain. Often, women are forced to get off the corporate ladder to welcome children and care for families. A woman's limited years of fertility and her female frame can also edge in on her ability to excel in athletics and physical roles that also require vigor and youth. Yet we are made to feel inadequate if we can't compete.

To succeed in these areas, women are forced to trade, or at least delay, natural childbearing and rearing to achieve success. When the female body must be manipulated by the demands of society to attain a goal that is at odds with its very nature, a dichotomy in the female psyche is created. Women are then at odds with their own bodies, and with men. This paradox destroys that which is innate and beautiful in the performance of healthy women's bodies and what should be a special interplay between the sexes.

In order for women to experience wholistic integration, women must be able to define success and accomplishment in accord with their innate female reality. Society's young adolescent girls should not expect their bodies to act like their male peers, nor should they be expected to ignore the obvious differences between male and female bodies. We do our daughters no favors when we acquiescence to a system where boys can move in upon female spaces and dominate us.

We need to work with men to bring a healthy respect and celebration of our differences, in light of our shared humanity and desire for mutually meaningful and healthy lives. Men are not the enemy of women's success. I know for certain that my husband has helped me to grow in respect for myself and has also done this for our three daughters. Loving husbands and fathers do so much to stabilize society and create space where women can be themselves. When men recognize the gifts of women and uplift them, and when women do not feel threatened by men's abilities, we can enjoy how we complement and elevate one another.

Because fertility is actually a shared function, men should be held to a standard where respecting our natural female cycles of fertility is the norm, but that requires us to communicate about our bodies with them. Men should not be seen as, nor treated simply as sperm donors, but seen in their fullness as human beings gifted with their own unique personalities and traits. If we want to be treated as whole and integrated beings, we owe men the same courtesy and we must bring them into the conversation about how we can improve the situation for all humans in need. We have to believe they can handle the truth about how we were created and partner with us. We women are the only ones who can tell them.

PARTNERS, NOT PREDATORS

Men are not the enemy of women and feminism. We need to acknowledge the many contributions of good men and highlight the sometimes-forgotten complementary relationship we must have with men to build up a fair and just society for all humans. We owe it to our sons to heal our trust issues with men.

As women, we must recognize we cannot understand the fullness of our female biological and spiritual capacities without looking at how our bodies interact with men's bodies. Our complementary bodies tell each other about how our bodies are supposed to work. They don't make sense on their own. There is no purpose to a vagina or uterus without a man's penis and sperm. It's not degrading to understand the purpose of our bodies–it's liberating!

We need to be able to see the human body in both forms and see that there is purpose and goodness there. To understand the fullness of the female body, it's imperative we understand the male body as its equal opposite. We require the opposite sex to define our own sex. In other words, we are given clues to our own identities and purposes merely by looking at our biological sex and saying it is different from the other, yet meant to work with the other.

Feminism has all too often ignored the important role of men in building an equitable society. Instead of the partners they must be, men are painted as offenders to women's dignity as potential abusers and rapists. It has become normal for feminists to refer to masculinity as "toxic" and to advocate for traditionally masculine stereotypes and activities such as sports and hunting to be avoided with young boys. There is a fear that by acknowledging a boy's maleness, he will grow to become a man who uses his strength and power to dominate women.

This can, and sadly does, happen when boys are taught strict male/female dichotomies and are told that boys can have only masculine attributes. But in my experience, I have seen that boys who are raised with a healthy sense of their difference from girls, and who understand that both boys and girls will each have some elements of masculine and feminine qualities, will take up the role of protector and defender for women later in their life. Boys who understand that having some feminine traits is normal and who are taught to understand their emotions do not feel a need to overexert masculine traits.

Children must be taught the deeper meaning of the male/female difference beyond shallow gender stereotypes in order to have a full understanding of their sexual realities and have an integrated identity. It is good for our sons and daughters to understand that they are different from each other but that they are also alike in many ways.

Different does not mean unequal in dignity, worth, and purpose, but it does mean that the purpose of their lives as either a male or female can be made clear by observing the reality of their physical bodies. As the two variations of the human form, both men and women lay equal claim to the dignity that must be afforded to all humans. Our sex, our race, our age, our health, and our positions in society should never be determinants of one human's worth over another.

GENDER STEREOTYPES

It is easy for us to get confused about the goodness and purpose of our bodies when we grow up being told our natural bodies should have no bearing or effect on our lives. It is easy for our young people to become confused about their identities and to feel disconnected from their bodies when we provide stereotypes of female/male to define themselves by that have little to nothing to do with their physical bodies.

When being a girl means simply preferring pink to blue, or being a boy means enjoying athletics instead of music or theater, we do our children a severe injustice. When we neglect to tell our children about the unique beauty of their bodies and instead define their identities on the whimsy of childhood preference, we set up our children to reject the amazing bodies they were created with.

We need not be so rigid with our surface definitions and expectations of male and female and gender. We must recognize that a boy can like pink or have long hair without him becoming a girl. His preference for things stereotyped as female does not make it necessary to unnaturally alter his body to appear to be more female. And a girl should be able to appreciate sports and excel at math and science without being treated as if she's stepping beyond the accepted norms. Our daughters should never feel guilty for being more than pretty faces.

The significance of being created either a boy or a girl lies in the unique contributions of our physical bodies. When our children can understand that their bodies point them to much deeper meaning than just liking certain colors or activities, they will find their lives more filled with purpose and direction.

The magic formula for female success is not in altering our natural bodies to be more male. It lies in our relationships with men who are willing to support and cooperate with us as equals, and who do not insist we acquiescence to their needs before our own.

IMAGINE IF

Now, for a moment, dream with me about what it would look like for a woman to live in a society that allowed us to create the rules for success in line with our biological reality....

Can you imagine if it was normal for women to have "red tent" days? What would it be like to have a workplace where it was standard for women to take the first two or three days of their monthly menstrual cycle off of work? We all know that our hormones make it difficult to concentrate and our productivity is compromised while menstruating, but the idea of acknowledging this truth is so radical in our current culture that most women cannot even let their minds wander into this territory.

We immediately begin to think about how embarrassing it would be to tell our boss when we have our periods…and then think about how we couldn't possibly ask for the luxury to rest our bodies…. But why? Because we have internalized deep shame about our female bodies. We are too embarrassed of what we perceive as a weakness, a liability to our success that we ignore the cramps, the bleeding, the fatigue, and pretend as if everything were great. It is not a weakness to need rest. I am certain men would insist on it if they bled for five days each month.

Think of nursing and working mothers, trying to fit breast pumping into the flow of the workday, in a cramped space, hidden away from her coworkers. Although we've made huge strides in normalizing this in our current culture, I still hear from women frequently who are embarrassed to store their milk in the staff refrigerator because someone keeps moving it out to the counter beside the fridge. One woman even shared with me that there was a note next to her milk with the word "disgusting" written on it. Talk about shaming a woman's natural body and its abilities.

It's no wonder that women are choosing to take massive doses of artificial hormones to suppress their fertility, sometimes only experiencing one cycle of bleeding per year. Or that they are forgoing trying to get pregnant until their late thirties, when their fertility is steeply declining. We've accepted that our bodies are an inconvenience because we've accepted male bodies, with their steady hormone levels as the ideal. We believe, subconsciously, that our female bodies are the problem, and we feel shameful of them.

When women make decisions to alter, suppress, and destroy their natural functions and deny their abilities to create, carry, and sustain new life, there is an internal fallout. We must intuitively protect ourselves emotionally and psychologically from the disintegration we are feeling. We are forced to compartmentalize and subsequently justify our decisions with false narratives.

We often fail to recognize the outside influences of shame in our decision-making process. We ignore the needs of our bodies and deny them the care they deserve. Ladies, this denial is serious. It must be addressed, but it is no small task. Women must be built up, empowered, and helped to understand their true and innate feminine abilities, abilities that are beautiful strengths, not hindrances.

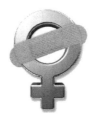

CHAPTER FIVE
YOUR BODY IS NOT THE PROBLEM

"Mother Nature usually wins in the end;
and Mother Nature is not a feminist."
CAMILLE PAGLIA, FEMINIST SCHOLAR

I began working with pregnant and breastfeeding women as a lactation professional in 2010. First as an intern at a local Women Infant Children (WIC) government office, then in labor and delivery at a small rural hospital, and finally in my own private practice. A large portion of the conversations I had with women transitioning into physical motherhood for the first time were spent reminding them over and over again they could trust their bodies to do what they were made to do. Many women are filled with so much fear and distrust of the labor and delivery process and lactation that they have almost convinced themselves to not even attempt natural deliveries or breastfeeding. Why are we so afraid of trusting our own bodies?

Women's doubt or distrust of their own bodies can lead to negative decisions concerning their health and the health of their children. Despite generations of feminists working tirelessly to empower women, many still lack authentic confidence. This lack of confidence stems from a disconnect due to countless conflicting messages about her body and the struggle of reconciling them with her own experiences.

Women have lost touch with how their bodies should act when healthy and have come to fear the very natural and uniquely feminine abilities to ovulate, gestate, and lactate. The number of times I have had women say to me, "Well, I could never give birth vaginally; my hips are too narrow" or "I'm sure I won't be able to breastfeed. My body never works right" are far too many. They have defeated themselves before even trying.

It's no wonder women doubt their bodies' natural abilities when culture provides every reason to doubt it. Our current women's health practices are contributing to a deep-seated mistrust and fear of how our bodies will perform when unsuppressed. We're afraid of how our natural bodies will work. Our culture favors women's bodies that are tightly monitored and controlled and leaves little room for women to get to truly know themselves and their abilities. It's time to address the fact that current cultural messages about women's bodies do not encourage women to make decisions that take their bodies' natural functions into consideration. Practices that suppress healthy functioning in women only perpetuate and reinforce the belief in women's inherent inferiority.

MALE-NORMED WOMEN'S HEALTHCARE

As we discussed in the previous chapter, we have adopted a male-normative culture and expect women's bodies to behave like men's and use drugs and devices to "fix" the problems our natural bodies present, such as fertility, pregnancies, and breastfeeding. I'm here to tell you—our female bodies are not the problem. Expecting them to act like men's bodies is the problem!

Who never gets pregnant after having sex?

Men.

Who never nurses a baby or requires lactation rooms for pumping while at work?

Men.

Who can go back to work immediately after becoming a parent and not bleed for weeks?

Men.

If sex no longer equals babies (like it doesn't for men), then women really don't need all the following support for pregnancy and parenting. It's "easier for everyone" (meaning society and the workplace) if women's bodies didn't demand anything more than men's bodies. We can see the evolution of women's healthcare over the past hundred years by looking at the women's movement and its acceptance of the male body as the ideal of health and success.

CONTROLLING MOTHER NATURE

We also see the masculine tendency to dominate and control nature in each area of healthcare as it relates to our feminine abilities. It is at the core of man to assert power and control over nature. Since the dawn of creation, man has endeavored to harness the power of and rule over the natural world. Man seeks to understand the laws of nature so as to dominate it. This has been used for great good as civilizations have risen through farming and industrialization. It is not a bad thing when properly applied. However, when directed at women, it often seeks to overpower and subjugate them. Women are different and that difference seems to make some men uncomfortable.

The female body has a much deeper and sacred understanding of the power of Mother Nature over us all. Since the beginning, fertility, new life, and death have been constantly present in the subconscious awareness of all women. Because of the nature of our menstrual cycles, their ties to the gravitational pulls on the earth, we have a stronger, more innate connection to Mother Nature and the reality of our fragile existence than men do. Our bodies remind us monthly of the possibility for new life, and then of the painful shedding and renewing of the sacred space within us when life is not conceived. We stand at the threshold of death when we deliver our babies. We can sense how delicate life truly is when we ponder our fertility.

For a new life to be nourished and grown, the protective mechanisms all have to be perfectly aligned and in balance, not only physically, but spiritually and emotionally as well. Our capacity to be fertile and multiply beyond ourselves is about surrender, acceptance, and trust. We must trust that our bodies will be able to do what they were created for and not kill us in the process. It is something that men will never be able to fully understand, not because they lack empathetic capacity, but because their natural bodies will never experience the total surrender that women submit to every month.

Our female bodies are built for an acceptance that men naturally rail and fight against. Mother Nature is something men feel capable of overcoming, while the truly wise woman understands that nature, and the Creator of nature, are always in control. When we get in the way in the processes of reproduction, we are truly in over our heads and often mess things up in our attempts to control what is happening. This is especially true in fertility, childbirth, and breastfeeding. We sabotage ourselves and throw the entire natural equilibrium out of orbit with healthcare practices that fail to cede control to nature and its processes.

For example, according to Diane Weissinger, MS, IBCLC:

> The delivery room procedures of most hospitals unwittingly work to undermine breastfeeding long before the baby takes its first breath…. In every mammal species…mothers who are deprived of their chosen place, time and sensations during the birth process have difficulty bonding and breastfeeding. Mammal bonding is adversely affected if birth is too hard – and if birth is too easy…Mothers in our culture haven't given birth since the early part of the 20th century. And no mammal who has birth taken from her goes on to nurse easily, or even to mother easily. It's not the breastfeeding that's the problem. It's the birth![1]

We fix things for convenience, to the point of destroying them.

WHAT ARE WE REALLY FIXING?

As women, we have learned to look for answers to the anxieties we feel about our bodies from everywhere except from within. As much as we want to deny it as feminists, we've adopted a victim status as women, and we depend on outside authorities to "fix" things that were never wrong with us to begin with.

We "need" pills to manage our natural fertility, or rather alter and suppress it. We insist on epidurals and cesarean sections before we've ever even leaned into the waves of our natural uterine contractions. We turn to artificial infant formula before our milk has even fully come in because we just don't think we can do it. We think we're broken, or not good enough to do what our bodies were made to do.

This is one of the greatest reasons we must abandon the old narrative of feminist thought as previous waves have said we need the drugs and devices of mankind to save us. We may feel like we're in control because we've demanded these things be given to us, but we've fallen for the lies of powerful companies and men who have convinced us we should be outraged if these things are withheld from us. In reality, if we look at who benefits most from these solutions, we will find it is often not women; it is the men who are content to use women's drive for success against them.

Recognizing the voices of authority in our culture that spread this worldview of bodily inferiority is the first step toward correcting it. The two places it is most obvious are in academia and medicine.

ACADEMIA AND WOMEN'S HEALTH

My first degree was in the field of psychology. As I reflect on my undergraduate experience, I realize that even with a college degree, which included several classes on human nature and relationships, I learned very little practical information about becoming a wife and mother. As a young mother living on a college campus, I felt very unprepared for the life I then lived. I wasn't equipped to integrate my education into a life plan that made me feel healthy and whole.

But instead of reaching back into my college textbooks and lecture notes for advice, everything I needed to know about understanding my mind and body and their effect on my behavior toward my family was coming from experienced mothers outside the campus setting. It wasn't intellectual or theoretical; it was real life.

I was struck by how unprepared I was to be a wife and a mother given that I had taken courses entitled The Biology of Women, Human Development, and even one class called Psychology of Marriage & Family. I felt wholly unprepared to navigate my biology, my growing newborn, and my new marriage and family after completing courses on these exact topics! The information fed to me as an undergraduate was not practical and had very little application to my life as a young mother. The curriculum fit a theoretical life that was not my reality and had more political slant than practical information.

Feminism says your body is inconsequential to your life experience. The women's movement used healthcare as a vehicle to accomplish a world where women no longer had female needs, and then used academia to convince us that biology must be overcome to find fulfilment. There was a very active women's studies department on campus with several prominent feminist professors, yet it seemed that when feminism and women's health intersected it was for the primary purpose of preventing motherhood, not supporting it. The sad conclusion was they weren't going to help me transition into motherhood.

MS. EDUCATION (OR MISEDUCATION)

The science course I had taken entitled The Biology of Women spent an entire semester discussing birth control practices across different cultures. There was nothing in that entire course explaining the natural cycles of fertility and infertility in women's bodies or how to recognize them. It didn't mention pregnancy beyond mentioning the possibility for unplanned pregnancies without proper contraception.

It focused heavily on the unequal burden childbearing places on women, yet never talked about childbirth and the drastic differences in maternal outcomes around the world. It didn't argue for the advancement of maternal and infant medical care to address high mortality rates. Nor did it acknowledge growing rates of infertility and other health challenges women face such as anemia. The theme of the class could easily be summed up by the phrase "women need birth control." That's it. That was the entire take-away from a semester-long class on women's biology with little to no opportunity for discussion or assessment about what women might truly need and want for biological health. Information was fed to us in a vacuum of women's rights but didn't address the right for us to care and fight for our uniquely female biology.

The attitude of the university regarding women's rights to be mothers was evidenced in many ways: by the lack of a lactation space on campus, nonexistent changing tables in the bathrooms, no on campus childcare for students, and no coverage for prenatal care in the student health insurance plan. The only women's health services at the student health center were pelvic exams, STI testing, and birth control prescriptions. Nothing for female students who wanted to learn about their fertility, support pregnancies, or breastfeed their babies.

WE NEED MORE

It was while living in this in-between place of college life and family life that I first understood the limiting nature of what has been defined as "women's health." At the time, I didn't understand the women's movement's role in the definition, but I understood that things were just not adding up to a comprehensive definition of the services I now needed as a woman. I began understanding that "women's health" had more to do with politics and the agendas of powerful organizations than the needs of the average woman's body.

The common definition of "women's health" in the United States for several decades has referred solely to reproductive systems and the management (most often the suppression) of women's fertility. This links directly back to the core problem of feminism being a dissociation from the biological reality of being female. Our fertility became a liability to the goals and lives women wanted to live because the women's movement failed to first insist our progress be made with full autonomy as women.

Motherhood became a liability to the progress women were making in the workforce, and so the idea that our fertility was a liability to our success and our "health" caught on like wildfire. Healthcare providers were recruited to further this worldview to the detriment of authentic women's healthcare needs.

The narrow focus of women's healthcare and overemphasis on our reproductive systems has limited the scope of medical advancements women truly need to understand the unique ways diseases affect the female body. The World Health Organization considers this excessive focus on reproductive health as a barrier to ensuring access to good quality healthcare for all women.[2]

I was realizing firsthand that the types of services I needed as a woman, a mother, were not included in a "women's health" platform. I couldn't find the care I needed in the university setting because someone, somewhere decided that higher education and babies didn't go together. "Having children while still living on a college campus didn't fit with the definition of what was considered healthy for young women, even though women in their twenties statistically have fewer negative outcomes for pregnancy and childbirth than women older or younger than them."[3] Unfortunately, the reason for the narrow scope of services in women's health has to do with the influence of the women's movement on our government and the millions of dollars spent managing women's bodies.

MONEY TALKS

For about a hundred years in the United States, we have been living with a view of women's healthcare that is neither healthy nor caring. It is based upon several flawed assumptions that have each taken center stage at different points in the women's movement:

- women are incapable of naturally managing their fertility
- childbirth is inherently dangerous
- women will be held back because of their motherhood

Many of these ideas have been to the benefit of drug companies and medical providers pushing their products and procedures on women.

Who benefits financially from women not understanding their fertility and therefore defaulting to artificial contraception?

Big Pharma and the providers writing the prescriptions for these drugs.

Who benefits when a woman fears the pain of childbirth and opts for every possible pain medication and intervention available?

The hospital and provider.

Who benefits when a woman opts not to even attempt breastfeeding and uses formula for her baby?

You guessed it, Big Business with deep marketing and sales budgets.

No one makes money on women's bodies doing their natural things without support or intervention, which the majority of women's bodies will do when healthy and properly supported.

Of course, there are obvious places in modern women's healthcare for practices that support our feminine abilities by means that are extraordinary. This is not a black and white issue (no pun intended, as racial disparity in women's health IS a major issue). For example, hormonal supplementation in pregnancy absolutely saves lives. Cesarean sections absolutely save lives. Artificial milk-replacement formula absolutely saves lives. Women with a history of trauma, mental health challenges, or even postpartum depression absolutely benefit from medical intervention for childbirth, recovery, and even formula to feed their babies.

These measures have their proper place; however, all women's health practices should be complementary to how the body would operate in full health. Women's health priorities must always communicate to women that they are strong, smart, and capable of working with their bodies. The goal for women's health should be a narrative saying under ideal circumstances, women's bodies will function in full health, free of disease and intervention, unsuppressed by artificial means. We should define the norm for women's healthcare not from the exception, but by the norm. We must consider how to have a complete picture of health, mind/body/spirit, and not sacrifice one for the benefit of another.

THE BODY IS **GOOD**, ALL OF IT, ALL THE TIME

We are gaining a greater awareness of the mind/body/spirit connection for health, but ironically, we often miss the connection between the feminine abilities of the body (ovulation, gestation, lactation) in optimizing women's health. As quoted earlier in this chapter by lactation consultant Diane Weissinger, how we birth affects how we breastfeed. And how we breastfeed affects our fertility.

The feminine abilities are connected, yet we miss the associations between hormonal surges and treat ability in isolation, meaning, oftentimes, we'll consider that one of the natural abilities is more special or important than the others and not work to advance healthcare that protects all three. There is a nonsensical segmentation with our feminine abilities and inconsistent acceptance of all women's naturally occurring functions.

We can see this in the birth community where many midwives and lactation consultants are in support of breastfeeding and will also promote natural childbirth because of the known risks associated with artificial labor augmentation and lactation failure.[4] However, very few seem to care about the risks associated with artificial hormonal contraceptives and their connection to low milk supply.[5] They will support gestation and lactation but are unwilling to fully embrace a woman's natural fertility, even when there are known risks to lactation from suppressing fertility.

In contradiction to the birth community, we have many churches and organized religions that embrace natural fertility but often ignore natural childbirth and breastfeeding. It is inconsistent and unreasonable. When we look at the main promoters of natural fertility in our country, mainly the Catholic Church, we see an almost inverse promotion of the natural abilities when compared to the birthing community.

A lot of effort will be put into promoting and supporting the creation of Natural Family Planning and Fertility Awareness Based Methods, as these methods have proven to be just as effective as artificial contraceptives in delaying pregnancy,[6] but these churches are often unwilling to even state that women's bodies are also capable of naturally birthing and breastfeeding their babies after they naturally conceived them. They stay far away from the natural birth and breastfeeding communities and often fail to give women a comprehensive theology of how the female body was created to function.

But perhaps the most ironic dissonance within current healthcare practices is the current push from some to embrace a strongly pro-contraceptive and pro-abortion position, while at the same time promoting natural childbirth. The creation of "abortion doula" groups as promoted by The Doula Project and other natural childbirth support groups,[7] and the bizarre combination of abortion clinics with birth centers clearly highlights the conflict that is happening within the field of women's healthcare.[8,9]

Either pregnancy is a beautiful, miraculous thing that the body is capable of achieving, or it is not and can be destroyed without second thought. They say that pregnancy and childbirth is healthy and empowering, and then they also say that it is healthy and empowering to destroy pregnancy in the same location. This inconsistency creates cognitive dissonance and further builds on the obviously confusing definition of what is healthy. Unfortunately, as modern women, we must wade through this conflict in our healthcare field every day.

FEMALE BODIES, WHOLE AND UNITED

Each of the feminine abilities has been embraced at some point in the history of the women's movement, but there has not yet come a time when ALL three feminine abilities have been accepted and promoted as the norm for women's health.

Feminism has had an especially fragmented relationship with women's natural bodies. The rhetoric has been confusing and inconsistent. "My Body, My Choice!" contrasted with "My Body, My Baby, My Birth Choice!" Or how about "Abortion on demand and without apology" alongside "Breastfeeding rights are human rights." There are so many mixed messages about what women want.

What women want should not be the only guideline for what women's healthcare is defined as. There should be objective standards of what is healthy.

Instead of all the differing opinions guiding our definitions, perhaps we should consider what is objectively good, and true, and beautiful (which our natural female bodies ARE). Surprisingly, with all the mixed and confusing messages being spoken about our bodies and our rights, very few seem to be consistently saying, "My natural body is not a problem, and ALL of me deserves to be in my original state, natural and unaltered." Or "True feminism protects and supports all of the natural functions of women's bodies." A culture that says it's acceptable for women to destroy themselves is a culture steeped in misogyny.

Our female bodies speak to us its purpose by how it acts when healthy, and many women will find peace and happiness when they know they are working with their bodies to achieve their dreams and goals. The definition of women's health must also include an awareness of mental health and female identity outside of just their physical productivity, but we cannot so broadly define women's health as to lose sight of the uniquely female body as the recipient of the care. They must work together.

When our bodies are unwell, our minds will suffer, and vice versa. We should receive mental healthcare that recognizes the effects of our bodies/hormones on our minds. We can't throw out the body. It matters tremendously, and everything that a woman's body is equipped to naturally do should be viewed as good.

DEFINING "HEALTH"

There have been many attempts to define women's healthcare, though political ties to feminist rhetoric often get in the way of actually using the naturally occurring functions of healthy women's bodies to define the norm. We know for women to experience the feeling of being healthy, it takes more than just her physical health being optimized; it includes her mind, her emotions, her environment, her relationships, and her sense of safety and stability.

However, in medicine, where the body is of primary concern when considering the health of women, there has been a trend to look the other way when the body is unwell and instead focus on other aspects of overall health. Consider this definition of "women's health" as defined in the *Canadian Medical Association Journal*, by Dr. Susan Philips, MD, CCFP. Note the obvious shift away from a biomedical definition of health and a broadening concept that focuses on social well-being.

> Women's health involves women's emotional, social, cultural, spiritual, and physical well-being, and is determined by the social, political, cultural, and economic context of women's lives, as well as by biology. This definition recognizes the validity of women's life experiences, and women's own beliefs about and experiences of, health. Every woman should be provided with the opportunity to achieve, sustain, and maintain health, as defined by the woman herself, to her full potential.[10]

This broadened definition acknowledges that holistic health is multilayered and takes into consideration women's relational needs. However, it also provides a dangerous opening for culture, society, and men to insert their influence by pressuring women's views of their own bodies. By failing to define how a female body should experience health as a biomedical function, we allow a definition of health that deviates from physical biological health. When this happens, all that becomes necessary for one to be healthy is to feel as though they meet the expectations of their given society.

DANGEROUS DEFINITIONS OF HEALTH

This broadened definition has the capacity to also justify the subjugation of physical bodily health to perceived personal mental or emotional well-being. Focusing on mental health over physical health allows us to support practices that run contrary to how every natural task of the body would normally function under the pretense of decreasing mental anxiety in women. This definition is the natural evolution of a movement that has been based upon a false notion of the equality of the sexes and one that has become more ideological than practical.

Third-wave feminism's key goals of self-identity and life experiences as key to happiness and health are obvious in this definition of women's health. The framework of this definition only works for incredibly privileged women in societies permeated with Christian ethics and fails women who are in cultural settings that expect gross mutilation and subjugation of the female body for her social acceptance.

Think for example of the more than 200 million women living in Africa, the Middle East, and parts of Asia who have undergone female genital mutilation (FGM).[11] Think of a young eight-year-old girl living in a village where the standard for women's health involves FGM. It could be argued using Philip's definition of women's health that her "health" is improved because she is accepted by her village. She has had her clitoris, labia minora, and majora scrapped off, her vagina cauterized, and her labial stumps stitched crudely together. Her future marriageability and social standing are now safe, thus assuring that the *social, political, cultural, and economic context* of her health aligns with accepted norms and expectations. Her own beliefs about her health and sexuality will meld with those of her community, and she will not experience mental anxiety about her place in society. And when she dies of infections to her mutilated genitals at the age of nine, her community will remember how good and "healthy" she was.

PATERNALISM IN HEALTHCARE

Ironically, even here in the United States, the field of women's health is often misogyny on full display. While we don't condone such barbaric practices as FGM, we do support fully the suppression and alteration of women's fertility, childbearing, and breastfeeding abilities every day through chemical and cultural mutilation of our bodies and motherhood.

The healthcare industry often displays flagrant disregard for the natural functions of women's bodies. The rhythms and hormonal cycles that evolve throughout a woman's lifespan are routinely manipulated, both surgically and pharmacologically.

Many women report being talked down to and made to feel embarrassed or ashamed when they talk to their doctors about their desires to take a more natural approach. It is a physician's responsibility to make sure their patients are informed about medications, procedures, and pathology so the patient is able to fully exercise bodily autonomy. Autonomy means that patients are free to make decisions in their perceived own best interest and that they are able to refuse medical care or treatment.

Paternalism is the greatest threat to this personal liberty of bodily autonomy in which we see a "big brother" sort of situation unfold. It is the intentional limitation of the autonomy of one person by another person.[12] This is usually done when a practitioner assumes a role of superior knowledge and authority and withholds information from a patient because they do not believe in their ability to make a decision toward good health. Women are treated as incapable of understanding their bodies, but in reality, perhaps it is the providers who are limited in this area.

Few providers in the healthcare industry understand the normal, natural functions of fertility and believe the altered state is the ideal for health. The CDC estimates that 65 percent of women of childbearing age suppress their fertility using hormonal contraception.[13] However, while the vast majority of women are suppressing their fertility, it's estimated that only 3 to 6 percent of physicians have accurate knowledge about the effectiveness rates of fertility awareness-based methods of family planning or know how to even observe signs of fertility.[14]

Female hormones and bodily functions are routinely altered to make women's bodies fit a societal expectation, not necessarily of optimal natural health, but rather, of accepted behavior and convenience to providers who don't know how to care for them otherwise. Much like those countries that insist FGM is in the best interest of their women's health, US medical standards insist that women's bodies should be controlled for their best interest as well. Paternalism in women's health is alive and well.

HANDMAIDS OR WARRIORS?

The autonomy of women to experience their natural bodies has been taken away because of some preconceived, accepted notion among the medical community and society that women are not capable of understanding or managing the issues of their natural fertility and natural childbirth. The number of times I have had physicians, healthcare workers, WIC staff, and public health nurses ask about my birth control method or birth choices, and then go on to lecture me about how poor my decisions are, is beyond my ability to count.

As I have become more educated and put more effort into understanding and respecting my body's abilities, I have been lectured and viewed as a problem patient for not following along with the current prescribed norms for women's health. Our government, along with many of our doctors, is currently promoting the idea that we are better off suppressing women's bodies than understanding them. In a climate pushing the use of universal birth control and hospitalized childbirth, there seems to be very little respect for the bodily and personal autonomy of women.

When women want to embrace their natural bodies, they are often accused of supporting the patriarchy by surrendering to male expectations for them to produce offspring. They are told they are weak-minded and traitors to the feminist cause, maternalists who just want women to be barefoot and pregnant.

In reality, it is the women who truly love their bodies and desire to learn about how they naturally work who are the most radical of all feminists. They refuse to conform to a male-normative culture that demands children be sacrificed for success and women's bodies be sacrificed for "self-actualization." These women refuse the nonsense that family planning is only a woman's issue and insist men be held accountable to their sexual urges and cooperate with women's cycles of fertility to attain responsible family planning.

They understand it is an undue responsibility for women to bear the entire weight of fertility when it is a shared function between men and women. These women desire healthcare that gives them solutions in line with their natural bodies and demand doctors provide them with solutions that do not destroy their healthy feminine functions. It is these women's voices that are needed to get the women's movement back on track and in line with our intended design.

It is time for us to hit the reset button on women's health, cultural expectations, and worldviews of women. We need to create a healthcare model that accepts and works with all of our uniquely feminine abilities and supports the truth of who we are as women.

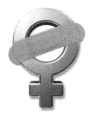

CHAPTER SIX

A NEW FEMINIST
MOVEMENT—WHOLISM

"The capacity to develop in a healthy manner, to regulate
stress, to balance emotions, and to feel for another human
being begins with mothers."

ERICA KOMISAR

Around 2005, I wrote a letter to the editor of the UMD student
newspaper. I'm not usually in the business of doing this, but I was so
shocked and disgusted by the image on a poster hanging up around
campus that I had to respond and voice my opinion. The image was of
a woman's naked crotch, her legs spread open, and her top half leaning
back, naked with breasts prominently displayed. It stopped at the neck
and didn't show her face. It was roughly drawn and not meant to be an
anatomical depiction but instead a crude advertisement for an event
hosted by a new student group calling itself FACE, which stood for

99

Feminists Advocating Change Etcetera. The image was supposed to be a rallying cry for women's rights.

The piece I wrote for the paper was titled, "That's Not My FACE," and it focused on the sheer absurdity of a group called FACE reducing a woman to only her genitalia. I pointed out that the obvious thing missing from the poster was, in fact, a woman's face and that these posters did the exact opposite of advocating for women's rights. They exploited and sexualized them with the adolescent drawing. I ended my short letter to the newspaper by saying,

> I cannot see any way in which these posters, or this talk, promote a better world for our daughters. They encourage a mentality that feminists have fought for years…that women are nothing more than sexual beings and objects. I am saddened by the turn modern feminism seems to have taken and can only hope that someday we will return to the logic of our feminist foremothers. Mary Wollstonecraft wrote in her "Vindication of the Rights of Women" in 1792, "considering women as a *whole*, let it be what it will, instead of a part of man, the inquiry is whether she have reason or not. If she has, she was not created merely to be the solace of man, and *the sexual should not destroy the human character*."[1]

These well-meaning student feminists had fallen for the exact lie that the first feminists in our country were refuting. By placing all of the visual attention on women's bodies, they ignored the importance of the whole identity of what it means to be a woman. Women have been viewed only as they relate to and serve the needs of men throughout time, which means we are often reduced down to a sexual purpose of quenching men's desire for pleasure.

When we ourselves place our identities only in our female genitalia, we do not create the sisterhood among women our feminine abilities have the power to. There is an essence of womanhood that is spiritual, sacred, and unique to women. It comes along with the physical functions of our female bodies, but it is deeper and more mystical. This essence of femininity could never be encapsulated with a crude drawing or any other visual display of the female body meant to astonish the viewer. And it certainly won't unite women to degrade ourselves for shock value.

For this reason, the current trend of wearing pussy hats and bumper stickers that say things such as "Vote Vaginas" have no place in the furthering of feminism. As if having a vagina means we automatically think synchronously. We must be very aware of the ways we currently are reducing women to mere genitalia by showcasing our sacred spaces and removing the mystique that surrounds the experience of the feminine.

We are bonded to one another by much more than our similar anatomy. We cannot fall into defining ourselves as merely the physical counterpart to men. This alone does not demand the respect due women for all we are and experience. It is more than what our bodies contribute that gives us equal dignity and ownership of mankind's destiny.

Our identities are complex and rich. We play into and support a misogynistic thought process when we encourage the reduction of our female identities into either just our physical or just our spiritual/emotional essences. We are a beautiful combination of:

- our feminine minds, rich with emotive and empathic capacity
- our evolving bodies, which cycle through hormonal fluctuations each month
- our spirits, which instinctively embrace the "others," the vulnerable and weak

To ignore the mind and spirit and define ourselves by merely our bodies is a painful dissection that robs our world of the female contribution to society. And on the flip side, if we reject our female bodies in favor of adopting a masculine spirit that mirrors patriarchy, we lose all the swaying, moving surrender that comes with the female experience. Reductionism is a common practice in our culture and is the exact opposite of what we hope to accomplish in creating a wholistic feminist movement.

REDUCTIONISM VS. WHOLISM

We humans tend to break down, or reduce, ideas or physical materials into their smallest components to gain a better understanding of what we're dealing with. We take rocks and minerals and even living organisms and put them under the microscope to see if we can determine what exactly makes up the whole of the thing. It gives us a sense of power and superiority when we can look at the periodic table and say that we know all the elements that make up our physical world.

We understand biology at the cellular level, and we understand the chemistry involved in the making of pretty much every material on the planet. We've even ventured so far as to say that we now understand the particular matter of the human body so well that we can reproduce human beings outside of the normal and natural way we've reproduced ourselves since the beginning of our species.

We humans have become vain enough to believe that by reducing something down to its smallest building blocks, we can gain the knowledge needed to reassemble the thing back to its original whole. We think we can capture the essence of what something is, human beings included, by putting together all the parts to create a whole. But in order to truly understand a human person, our parts cannot be dealt with in isolation. We must see the whole person as interconnected at all times, especially if we want to bring health and wellness to a person. This includes the mind | body | spirit being treated with consideration for one another.

"Wholism" emphasizes the importance of the whole and the interdependence of its parts. In other words, to understand something, we must look at it in its entirety, and part of doing so is understanding the individual parts that make up that whole and how they relate to one another. Reductionism must be rejected, in healthcare especially, if the state of things for women is to be improved culturally. The whole is much greater than the sum of the parts, and we cannot be reduced to merely our parts.

WHOLISTIC HEALTH

As discussed in the previous chapter, defining health for women has been a sometimes-controversial topic. It has been narrowed and broadened erroneously to either look only at the body or to prioritize social and emotional factors over the body. We have discussed how the women's health field has never accepted all the physical functions of a woman's healthy fertile body in union with one another. In the same way it has also failed to provide a framework for how a healthy female human should be free to live in her body as a member of a healthy society, where her female mind and spirit is also accepted along with her physical body. We cannot consider health too narrowly by defining it only as the physical health of a person, but we cannot broaden it so far as to lose sight of the significance of the body entirely.

This long-standing connection between the mind, body, and spirit is not unique to women; men also need to have healthy integration of these three elements to be whole. Both men and women will feel unbalanced and unwell when one of these facets is suffering. For example, most, if not all, of us have observed that when we experience mental stress our heart starts to race.

"Constant worry and stress over jobs, finances, or other problems can cause tense muscles, pain, headaches, and stomach problems. It may also lead to high blood pressure or other serious problems."[2]

Our bodies can have effects on our minds and spirits as well.

"...pain or a health problem like heart disease can affect your emotions. You might become depressed, anxious, and stressed, which could affect how well you treat, manage, or cope with your illness."[3]

There is a unique challenge in the women's healthcare field at this time in history, as it has become routine and normal care for the fertility of the female body to be categorically rejected, and women's health reduced to primarily altering, suppressing, and destroying the natural reproductive system. The female mind and spirit will struggle when the female body is treated as inconsequential to identity and health.

This is why we must demand the norm for a healthy human, man or woman, to start with an unaltered reproductive system. The reproductive organs are just as much a part of us as the digestive system, and without them functioning in a healthy and optimized way, we are not whole.

THE BODY MATTERS

It is vitally important that when we talk about wholism and becoming self-integrated we accept the starting point as an acceptance of the physical reality before us. We need to see our bodies as outward signs, or clues, to the nature of the minds and spirits that reside within. Nature will always overcome and reset itself despite our meddling. We can either acknowledge that and work with it or continuously expend time and energy fighting against it. When we work in cooperation with nature and its laws, we will be whole and at peace because our energy can now be directed to becoming the best version of ourselves, as we truly are.

Without acknowledging first that our DNA, hormones, and physical stature impact the way we live in and interpret the world, we can't understand the cues given to us by the vessel that is truly ourselves. Our physical bodies teach us deep spiritual truths about who we are and what will bring us the greatest meaning and joy in life. We can't manipulate the mind | body | spirit connection without consequence. We need to work to create environments that allow each person to embrace first the physical body they were born with, and then encourage the expression of unique minds and spirits that accompany these bodies.

This is not to take lightly the problem of deeply flawed gender stereotyping happening in many cultures, but it is crucial for the health of both women and men that we stop allowing reductionism that says it is okay to separate the mind from the body and the spirit. We cannot dissect the human person and pit the mind | body | spirit against one another. It is not healthy for us to grossly alter a person's physical body to meet gender stereotypes for a given culture.

We cannot change the essence of a human person's identity by doing this; we only create the illusion of meeting a desired stereotype. When we do this, we create the situation where the mind | body | spirit are at odds with one another. When the mind does not match the physical body. there is discord. The internal dissonance between the will and nature can never be settled if they are at odds; a person who does not embrace the physical vessel of their identity will be constantly at war with oneself. The health of a human's mind, body, and spirit is meant to be in harmony with one another. When these are all in balance, a person experiences wholeness. When we allow one to rule over the others, the human person is not truly themselves but an unbalanced expression of their own reality.

LESSONS IN ILLNESS

For most people, there is a much less dramatic struggle that happens internally when the mind | body | spirit all want something different. We may not be aware of that struggle or an imbalance until we become sick in one area and are forced to stop to put things back in order.

Somewhat ironically, I came down with COVID-19 as I began writing this chapter. I struggled tremendously to listen to my body as it begged for rest, while my mind was watching my day planner and all the deadlines I had to meet with my editor and everyone else in my life. In some ways, it was a gift because I was forced to face the ways in which I was allowing my mind to overrule the needs of my body. I had to ask myself why I was doing this and realized I was reaching for a male-normed, high-productivity standard for my work.

I had to recognize that my hard-driving expectations for productivity were hindering my own recovery. I was placing high expectations on myself, where others were actually granting me room and grace to recover. My mind, body, and spirit were all in need of care, and this necessary pause was exactly what I needed to put me back in sync with myself.

In many ways, the pandemic put us all back in touch with the reality of nature and the immense power that tiny germs and viruses can have on us physically, socially, emotionally, and spiritually. Within a matter of a few short weeks, the entire world felt the effects of being socially distanced and isolated from one another. Many contracted the virus and experienced the effects of the physical illness. We were all cut off from our communities of faith and friendships that feed and sustain our souls. The toll on humanity collectively will play out for many years, as our health has been attacked on all fronts and our recovery will require a multifaceted approach.

Global pandemics are uncommon, and more often, we experience illness in only one facet of our health at a time. The struggle can spread into other areas of our health if prolonged, but usually we deal with one problem area at a time, such as addressing a broken leg by having it cast. However, we often fail to consider if a traumatic event, such as an accident that caused the broken bone, is also causing mental or spiritual illness. Our healthcare often falls short of fully healing people because it does not customarily check on the other facets of health. Wholistic healthcare is an approach that takes all of these things into account and treats the whole person mind | body | spirit.

Imagine a healthcare system that provides not only for all the physical needs of your body but also has mental and spiritual health services as well. What would it feel like if after receiving the care for the broken bone, you were invited to process the event with a trained mental health professional? Perhaps many people would not need that comprehensive care, but for those who are struggling, imagine how life-changing being fully seen would be? I regularly see the need for this complete care in many areas of women's healthcare; with new postpartum women falling through the cracks with inadequate postpartum depression screenings, with little to no chaplaincy services following infant loss and miscarriages, with the anxiety breastfeeding mothers face when they struggle to nurse. Oftentimes, we address the physical needs of the body but miss the hurting mind and spirit.

NEW AWARENESS OF TRAUMA

There is a growing body of evidence pointing toward wholistic care as a superior model for wellness. One of the most exciting advancements has been in the emerging field of trauma-informed care. In 2014, Bessel van der Kolk, a Boston-based Dutch psychiatrist and pioneering PTSD researcher, wrote a groundbreaking book called *The Body Keeps the Score: Brain, Mind, and Body in the Healing of Trauma*. In it, he talks about developments in the fields of neuroscience, developmental psychopathology, and interpersonal neurobiology, and states:

> Research from these new disciplines has revealed that trauma produces actual physiological changes, including a recalibration of the brain's alarm system, an increase in stress hormone activity, and alterations in the system that filters relevant information from irrelevant. We now know that trauma compromises the brain area that communicates the physical, embodied feeling of being alive. These changes explain why traumatized individuals become hypervigilant to threat at the expense of spontaneously engaging in their day-to-day lives. They also help us understand why traumatized people so often keep repeating the same problems and have such trouble learning from experience. We now know that their behaviors are not the result of moral

failings or signs of lack of willpower or bad character— they are caused by actual changes in the brain.[4]

The medical definition of trauma has long referred to damage or injury to the physical structure of the body, but with the evolution of our understanding, we can see that wellness can be affected by distressing and disturbing experiences as well. Sometimes these experiences involve our own physical injury, but they can also include threats to our safety or those we care about. Giving women the vocabulary to express the traumas that often go along with a paternalistic healthcare system is a huge step forward. Seeing the trauma many women experience and adjusting our practices to prevent it is critical.

HEALTHY MIND | BODY | SPIRIT

Let's dive in and look closer at how a healthy mind, body, and spirit operate. We'll look at each of them individually first, but remember, we can never separate them completely because each depends upon the others to function.

MIND

The mind is where we manage our emotions, our thoughts, our personality. It is where our memories of past experiences are held and is where our self-image and concept of the type of person we are comes from. Self-discipline, habits, and willpower come from the work of our minds. The mind is capable of reason and learning. We have control over our minds and can choose the path we want to walk.

With the practice of self-awareness and mindfulness, we can choose the emotional responses, daily habits, and viewpoints we have. What we tell ourselves about our talents and abilities will direct our actions, either positive or negative. Therefore, active management and awareness of deep subconscious self-perceptions is very important if we want to achieve a life of meaning and purpose.

The mind houses tremendous abilities and liabilities. Greater awareness of mindset limitations is becoming known, and even some school curriculums are being adjusted to promote growth mindsets in young children. The alternative mindset to a growth mindset is called a fixed mindset, where a failure confirms one's ability, and there is no further attempt to master a new skill. Fixed mindsets believe that qualities such as intelligence, athleticism, and character are fixed traits and that a person can't change. A common element of growth mindset curriculums is to add the word *yet* to the end of statements so that improvement and change become the expectation. "I can't read" becomes "I can't read, yet."

A well-trained mind is an incredible tool for living a life that is integrated, rich, and full of meaning and purpose. A healthy mind can overcome the psychological stress that comes with physical illness by choosing to value redemptive suffering. The ability to choose our mindset and worldview is too often misunderstood and overlooked.

Of course, there are physical factors that can affect the health of our minds. Because the mind/body/spirit are directly connected and interrelated, we need to remember that the physical home of the mind is within our bodies, more specifically our brains, and that it is subject to challenges from chemical imbalances and structural injuries.

Imagine you have a computer in your head that controls everything you do: **Your brain is the hardware—that's the physical box.** Your brain has all the power connections, wiring, storage, memory and processing power you need to function as a human being. **If**

your brain is the hardware, then your mind is the software. It's the operating system that gathers, stores and manages information, using the massive processing resources of your brain. In reality, your brain and your mind are inseparable—they're part of the same entity and one can't operate without the other.[5] — Caroline Ferguson

Caring for our minds includes careful monitoring of how well it is performing its function as our operating system. If we note we are feeling mentally sluggish, anxious, depressed, or confused, we should not hesitate to seek care for the body or the spirit that may be negatively affecting our minds.

Signs our minds are struggling:

- stress levels high
- anxiety/depression
- loneliness
- trouble organizing thoughts/schedule
- constantly overwhelmed
- can't focus, distracted often
- unsure of priorities

BODY

In general, our society still has a very distorted view of the body, women's bodies in particular. This makes it very difficult to assess objectively how our bodies are doing. All too often, women are told to fit a physical mold that allows for little individuality or variation. Objectification, body-shaming, and dangerous stereotyping pollute our world and ideas of health. Women must suppress and control their natural bodies in order to fit into the molds provided by society that supposedly lead to happiness and success.

All too often, women chip away at themselves, desperately trying to create themselves into the people the world asks them to be. A handful of statistics puts this into perspective:

- 91 percent of American women are unhappy with their bodies and resort to dieting.[6]
- 42 percent of American girls in 1st through 3rd grade want to be thinner.[7]
- Studies at Stanford University and the University of Massachusetts found that 70 percent of college women say they feel worse about their own looks after reading women's magazines.[8]

Around every corner, and at every milestone of their girlhood, women are belittled, body-shamed, and made victims of dangerous gender stereotyping. Girls are taught that their bodies are for looking "pretty" or "hot" and for gaining approval from others. They are taught that girls who match certain images are somehow better than those who don't. But the messages they receive about their bodies aren't limited to their physical appearance; girls also receive powerful messages about their roles and limitations they will likely experience living in a female body.

The body should serve as your primary guide to identity. We cannot cede to a definition of health that says it is acceptable to alter, suppress, or destroy a woman's body for her well-being. It is an attack on her and leaves her without the guide that her body is for understanding her whole identity. It's imperative that we know how a healthy female body should function because knowledge is empowering.

Along with supporting our uniquely female bodies and our feminine abilities, we must also recognize the basic needs for rest, exercise, a healthy diet, and good hygiene. Taking good care of our bodies supports our minds and our spirits, but it must be kept in proportion and not become an obsession.

When our bodies need rest, it would not be caring to force ourselves to go for a run. In a culture that values productivity, our bodies can be subjected to sleepless nights, high levels of stress hormones, and surgical and chemical alteration just to meet the expectation of society. Think of those in the entertainment industry who feel pressures to appear perpetually young as they age. We should not be expected to sacrifice our bodies' natural states for an unhealthy, unnatural, inauthentic standard.

Signs we need to care for our bodies:

- stiffness, pain, inflammation
- exercise and movement not a priority
- not eating well
- gaining/losing too much weight
- daily hygiene not a priority
- feeling constant fatigue

SPIRIT

The spirit, or the soul of a person, is an ancient, yet culturally relevant, concept. It refers to the human realization that there is something beyond ourselves, something greater that draws our heart toward a relational existence. It encompasses our desire to be in communion with that life-giving force—our God, our Creator. We seek something outside of ourselves that gives us meaning and purpose, the source of our commission. Having a deep acceptance that we are created a certain way for a specific reason helps us to understand and honor our talents and passions, and to accept our bodies as gifts capable of carrying us down the pathway that fully encompasses who we are.

Our spirits are our natural attraction to beauty, goodness, and truth. It is the part of us that is moved to tears when we hear a touching song, or when we witness a sunset that illuminates the skies with breathtaking beauty. When we feel a surge of goodness holding our newborn child, it is our spirits that are alive and speaking to us! It reminds us we are meant to live a life on fire with passion, purpose, and meaning. It makes us want to seek truth and possess all the applaudable human virtues that the saints and heroes had.

The spirit is the core of our integrated identity and directs what we should do with our lives. The mind manages our emotions and makes decisions toward following this path, and the body is the vehicle that will deliver us to our destination. But it is the spirit that is ultimately able to give us the sense of peace and inner wellness that comes with being whole.

There is strong evidence to suggest that a universal recognition of a Creator has existed in all civilizations throughout time. There seems to be a human default to religion; or perhaps a more apt way to express this tendency is to say that humans are wired to search for their origin and meaning. This longing is ingrained as we seek wholeness and completion. In knowing *whose* we are, we can know *who* we are.

We can sense when there are missing pieces in the puzzle and we move with deliberation, sometimes compulsively, toward finding those pieces so we can see the full picture. We desire to know ourselves; therefore, we desire to know our purpose and meaning. This is where our spirits can guide us.

We need to care for our spirits through intentional daily care. The spirit can be easily overtaken by the mind and body and pushed down.

When it is unwell, all of our gains in other arenas will feel hollow. Disintegrated.

Signs our spirits are suffering:

- feeling isolated and lonely
- not seeing or appreciating beauty
- disengaged from a faith community
- skepticism, pessimism, and despair about life
- lack of motivation to pray
- narcissism and self-centeredness

The spiritual facet of our identities is not defined simply as a religious belief or practice; it goes much deeper into our very essence. It speaks to the idea that each person is created as an individual and that they have a personality, a set of gifts, and a passion that makes them unique and irreplaceable. All humans possess a unique and irreplaceable spirit. As women, we share an even more precious bond as the feminine essence; the womanly spirit is built into the very nature of our bodies.

THE SACRED FEMININE

During my first years of motherhood, I got to know so many amazing women. I met these women at La Leche League meetings, mother exercise/stretching classes, hypnobirthing childbirth prep classes, and mother gatherings with dozens of women with babies snuggled safely in wraps sitting around a campfire sharing kombucha recipes. I know this all probably sounds a little "crunchy" and weird to some, but the connections and authentic friendships formed helped me to remember my own strength at times when I felt overwhelmed and burdened by my beautiful babies.

These women believed motherhood was a sacred gift and that sisterhood between mothers compelled women to support and lift up one another. It was an unlikely respite for my soul. It awakened my spirit to the good, the true, and the beautiful reality that women in community supporting one another is innate to feeling whole.

It was my relationships with these women that confirmed my beliefs about the future of the women's movement beginning with the acceptance of women's natural bodies as the guide to our collective female voice.

I was surrounded by this group of natural and fiercely authentic women who were very different from me ideologically, but who were totally united in support of me as I learned to birth and breastfeed my own babes. Their witness of embracing their female bodies fully inspired me to see myself in a more complete and valuable way. When I was exhausted and at a mental low, expecting baby number four in under five years, these women threw a blessingway celebration for me. Unlike a baby shower, these celebrations entail pampering, words of affirmation, postpartum meal organization, and so much more. It was exactly what I didn't realize I needed.

That pregnancy was hard. I had been enduring looks of exasperation from nurses and providers when I came in for my prenatal appointments with my toddlers in tow. After several semi-rude comments from nurses, and my own sheer exhaustion, I checked out from traditional prenatal care and decided to stay home and work with a midwife.

There was no judgment or snarky comments from the women at the mothering groups, only encouragement and affirmation that I was strong and healthy. They told me I could do hard things and built me up. It was as if they instinctively knew what I needed to hear when they each brought forward a blessing bead at my blessingway and pressed it into my hand with words of love. They conveyed complete confidence in my ability to bring my baby into the world. They told me the truth about who I was created to be and reminded me of my own strength.

They helped me string together all those beautiful beads into a labor necklace that I kept beside my birth tub and looked at when the strong waves of active labor kicked in. I remembered each woman and her words of assurance about my own abilities. They believed in me at a time when I was losing faith in myself and the medical community. They spoke to my feminine spirit and called it forward to guide me.

The more time I spent around these women the more I desired to use my own talents to turn around and help my sisters coming up behind me. I went back to school to become a women's health specialist because I knew that authentic women's healthcare and real feminism speaks truth and courage into women's hearts, not the judgment and exclusion I received when I spoke my mind. Real feminism should accept all of me, motherhood included. This is what I believed feminism to be as a child. I believed women could succeed with their babies at their side and that true feminists would fight for my right to do that.

The women I met and was surrounded by during those years were doing awesome things alongside raising their babes. These women were not giving up on dreams and aspirations because they had become mothers. Most of these women embraced lives that were totally different from the lives they lived prior to motherhood, but they were loving it. They seemed to be finding even greater inspiration and drive to contribute to society because of their babies.

One created a "women circling women" group that lifted up new mothers and encouraged them through their pregnancies and organized the blessingway celebrations for new moms. One mom ran a very successful Etsy store selling the cutest homemade baby leg warmers from her home. Another was a professional belly-dancing instructor who encouraged postpartum women to rebuild their core strength and self-appreciation through dance. There was an entire group of mothers who came together for group exercise and song and dance with their children and then organized community barn dances just to share joy! Their female bodies, their motherhood, had initiated relationships they would have otherwise not had, and it was incredibly hopeful to witness. They were alive and living out their motherhood to the benefit of our entire community.

NEED FOR COMMUNITY

Our bodies have been telling us a basic truth since the dawn of creation: we were made for relationship. The female body is the exact prototype for an honest, open, authentic relationship. It is always seeking relationship and is a physical reminder that we can either embrace others or reject them and close ourselves off. Our bodies open to envelope the "other" in sexual intercourse, our wombs welcome the "other" with the conception of a child, and our breasts nourish the "other" through lactation. We are naturally "other-oriented," and our female bodies are perfectly suited to teach man the deep truths about relationship. Our bodies can unite humanity or tear it apart through rejection and separation.

For the millions who carry pain and trauma in their histories, the need for mother-led community is even greater.

> "Social support is not the same as merely being in the presence of others. The critical issue is *reciprocity*: being truly heard and seen by the people around us, feeling that we are held in someone else's mind and heart. For our physiology to calm down, heal, and grow we need a visceral feeling of safety. No doctor can write a

prescription for friendship and love: These are complex and hard-earned capacities. You don't need a history of trauma to feel self-conscious and even panicked at a party with strangers—but trauma can turn the whole world into a gathering of aliens."[9] —Bessel van der Kolk

We as women excel in the healing art of receptivity and reciprocity. When we embrace the lessons our natural bodies point us toward and open our hearts to others, we can provide the acceptance and safety needed for healing. The core problems of modern feminism are a dissociation from the biological realities of our female bodies and a lack of recognition that we share this female experience of the body with all other women. Imagine the power of a feminist movement that promoted wholism—an integration of the mind, body, and spirit and recognition that we are all mothers to the world. Now is the time. Our physical bodies speak deep spiritual truths about the necessary role of women to bring peace to the human family. For the sake of humanity and its future, let us not ignore ourselves.

WHOLE IDENTITIES

We must be fully ourselves with a healthy mind | body | spirit in order for our unique creative capacities to flourish and for our true identities to come alive. When we dissect ourselves into little bits of who we fully are, we reduce our identities and our values to society by saying things like, "I'm just a stay-at-home mother." When we take on our careers or vocational states as our core identities, we do ourselves a huge injustice. When we forget all that makes up the whole of ourselves, we forget we are truly beautiful masterpieces capable of creating and sustaining life on earth.

Who we are as unique and irreplaceable human beings could never be summed up by our jobs, our outward appearances, or other classifications that could be surmised from observation. We are not only what we do. What we produce is valuable and speaks to our rich identities, but it does not begin to express the fullness of our being. The whole of our being as humans is incredibly complex, so beautifully compiled through our unique lived experiences, our families of origin, our places of birth, and the time in history that we've occupied a particular space. These are all the special ingredients that make up our spirits, our souls.

Suffice it to say, it is truly impossible for a human being to ever be cloned or created again. Even if your DNA were to be perfectly replicated, there could never be another you. The whole of you and me will never exist again in the history of the world. Every circumstance of your existence from conception to current time would need to be exactly replicated to create the human person you are, which is impossible. We each live our unique lives once, and the life we live can never be reduced to the sum of its parts.

Truly, the greatest question any human can ponder is ***what is the whole purpose of your life?*** All of it. Not just your career or your goals. What is it only you have been perfectly prepared for and equipped to contribute to our world? The world needs you to live it.

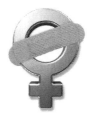

CHAPTER SEVEN

WOMEN'S SPACE IN THE WORLD

"It takes courage to grow up and be who you really are."
E. E. CUMMINGS

In a male-normed world where success looks like having a lot, doing a lot, and being widely respected, where are women who embrace their femininity going to thrive? Where do we fit in? Is there a place where women "belong," where our feminine gifts can shine, and where we are free to be fully ourselves? Do we belong in the home raising the next generation, or in the world? Each woman must be taught to navigate that question for herself, being accountable to her unique mind, body, and spirit.

Women have experienced a three-pronged attack on identity historically depicting our minds as weak, our bodies as burdens, and our spirits as inconsequentially ethereal. Along with widespread mutilation of our female fertility, the feminine spirit is also often crushed in a male-normed world. The unique creativity we each have can be stifled under heavy expectations for productivity and success.

I started this book with the premise that women are incredibly divided, generally unhappy, stressed out, and unsettled because we do not know who we are. We have lost our personal female identities and our collective voices as women because we've devalued our own unique minds, bodies, and spirits. We've allowed ourselves to be victims. We don't acknowledge or even see our need to be whole and healthy, so we operate while missing half of the information about ourselves. We're disjointed, reduced, and unfulfilled.

The women's movement pointed us off track by telling us we'd find greater fulfillment outside the home; never mind that each woman is unique and will have her own passions that bring her to life. Work in a traditional setting will be a great place for many of us to flourish, but for just as many of us, being present in the community, the home, and any other place we find ourselves will allow us to burst open with inspiration and originality. We'll talk more about that in the final chapter.

What connects us is not that our passions are the same, but that our bodies are connected in a deeply spiritual way by virtue of being women. We can't build a women's movement by making women all act the same, but rather we can and must build a new movement acknowledging we match one another in our *being*, not our doing. We need to carve out a place for all women to thrive by uniting around our sameness. We need to hold language and space that can serve as guides for women to discover their full identities and be whole.

REDUCTIONISM HURTS OURSELVES, AND OTHERS

Part of searching for personal health and identity is ultimately the quest to be seen and accepted as equal. If we struggle to value our own worth and feel accepted the way we were created, it can be tempting to create a persona to display the parts of us that get attention and feel seen.

One obvious temptation is to reduce ourselves to our bodies' outward appearances and sex appeal. We present ourselves in this superficial way believing this is where we can find our power. We hide our minds and adopt popular opinions in search of acceptance, reducing our personality to what we believe will bring us companionship. Sadly, sharing this shallow version of ourselves seems easier than revealing our intellect, voicing our opinions, or bearing our heart vulnerably to another and asking for their approval. Instead of being fully ourselves and forming authentic relationships, we accept the bare minimum that others present to us and reduce ourselves to those around us.

Nothing we do occurs in a vacuum. This exchange has effects on other people and society as a whole. We ultimately encourage a culture of surface-level interactions, yet treat them as deeply intimate, which furthers the notion that people are not complex human beings with real needs. What we may see as being empowered or a personal expression of our self is actually a reduction of ourselves and others to consumers of people as products.

The greatest threat currently to experiencing individual wholism is societal pressure to accept identities promoting our reduction through the separation of the mind | body | spirit connection. When this happens, we reduce ourselves down to merely a facet of who we are, thus confining us to the title we've chosen. We must always remember that who we truly are is not determined by what we do, but by who we are. Titles will always fall short of providing true meaning to life when they box us into a reduced identity, especially one that disregards the importance of the body.

WOMEN HAVE A RIGHT TO OUR SPACE

The body tells us a truth about reality. It alone gives us the first clues about purpose and identity, and that reality cannot be taken away from anyone. When we accept and promote titles at odds with this reality, we hurt others who are the legitimate owners of a title that is not our own. Even though we may not mean to hurt others, blurring the lines of reality affects everyone.

The body as a guide to reality matters when it comes to equality and making things fair, especially in situations of competition where women are seeking to excel and reach their highest potential. Just like most mammals, human males and females do have discernable differences in body composition and muscle mass. Our sexual dimorphism tells us scientifically that those with biological male attributes are going to have larger hearts and lungs and have taller bodies. Women will be approximately 50–60 percent as strong as men in the upper body, and 60–70 percent as strong in the lower body.[1]

Men and women are not equal to one another as competitors when placed beside one another on the track or basketball court. Biological males have an advantage in games of physical strength, speed, and endurance when competing against biological females. It is not discrimination to observe and note these differences. It is discrimination against women to ignore them, and even more so to insinuate that women speaking up in opposition are being unladylike or rude.

Most women I know are more than willing to welcome men into spaces of intimate friendship and will even advocate that men be welcome in traditionally female professions, such as teaching and becoming stay-at-home parents. Women are not trying to keep men out of female public spaces; however, men should appreciate and not abuse our goodwill toward them by recognizing that not all spaces should be open and available to them.

Women need the community of other women, as well as the encouragement and acceptance we can so graciously extend to others. However, our hospitality and propensity to accept and welcome others can be abused and has been in recent years by men infringing upon and moving into female spaces.

We have a right to safety and deserve space to relax so we can reach our fullest potential as women. Many women have experienced tremendous suffering and trauma at the hands of men. Allowing men into women's dressing rooms, bathrooms, or locker rooms leaves little room for these women to exist. When biological males are allowed into spaces that should be safe havens for women to commune with one another, the ability to relax is removed, and our natural feminine instinct to welcome and accept is used against us. Most women want to be nice, but at what point does our niceness result in our own voices being silenced?

It's not just physical spaces that men have moved into, it's our places of supposed honor as well. In 2015, Caitlyn Jenner, formerly known as Bruce Jenner, a world-class male Olympian was honored with the title "Woman of the Year" from *Glamour* magazine.[2] The honor was given to him for the apparent courage he displayed while undergoing radical body manipulation in a "sex change" surgery, and the bravery it took to come out looking like an attractive woman. A man, who has incredible privilege with his position and finances, was selected before millions of women who have spent their entire lives struggling to gain acceptance and accolades in a world he already excelled in.

It shouldn't be a surprise that a biological man can become woman of the year when our success as women is defined by our media and publications as nothing more than how sexually appealing we are to men. The reduction of women into personas that fit magazine headlines has been going on for a century. *Glamour* was founded in 1939 as a women's magazine and has focused heavily on fashion, beauty, and celebrity culture for all these years, evidently the true markers of womanhood. It seems that if someone can achieve all these things, then they must meet the criteria of a successful and admirable woman. I guess if that is all it takes, then congratulations Caitlyn Jenner. That is not an honor most women I know would find to be a fulfilling accomplishment.

Clearly it is women's spaces and honors that are infringed upon, not vice versa. One couldn't imagine a men's magazine choosing a woman transitioned to appear like a man being celebrated as "Man of the Year."

WE ARE MORE THAN OUR DESIRES

Ironically, if we truly believe that our gonads do not determine our sex, why do so many people spend so much money artificially recreating the genitals of the sex they desire to be? Not only does the Jenner story highlight the broken lens we view success for women as dependent upon our appearances, it also shows how the definition of sex moving away from the presence of biological markers has caused the terms *man* and *woman* to be muddled nearly beyond recognition.

Whereas sex has traditionally been declared at birth based upon the observation of external genitalia, now it has become trendy to declare that a parent cannot know the sex of their child until the child is old enough to tell the parent. This loss of guidance for our children in knowing their biological identities will lead to a false belief that our sex is indeed insignificant and that the body parts are changeable. We should fully expect future generations to accept gross bodily mutilations when we fail to tell them how beautiful and special they were created. We set our children up for lives that will leave their mind | body | spirit at odds with one another if we don't tell them the simple truth about who they are. It is not a threat to a child's identity to tell them that they were born a boy or a girl; it is the necessary generational guidance that every person needs to know their own story.

Perhaps we have arrived at this moment in time when so many of us are at odds with our own bodies because we no longer trust the Creator, or Mother Nature? Our spirits are clearly not well if we can so easily believe that we were not made with intention and love. Can we ever truly know who we are if we lack the knowledge of *whose* we are in the first place?

BREASTFEEDING OR CHESTFEEDING?

In my field of lactation care, I have watched as biological terms have been replaced by more politically correct words. Mothers are now referred to as "lactating parents," breastfeeding has been swapped out for the more gender-inclusive term "chestfeeding." The intention is to be inclusive and to open the lactation door to people who are experiencing body dysmorphia and gender confusion; however, when you open this door too widely, you lose the ability to care well for the women who truly need the help the most.

It is unhelpful for me as a care provider to use terms that conflict with scientifically correct terms and avoid calling a woman a mother. She IS a mother, and even if her sexual orientation or inner gender awareness are at odds with that, she still deserves that title. It is a relational term of the mother to her child and has historically been protected and revered. Having a strong cultural acceptance and expectation for the term assures she receives the respect and care she deserves, and also that the child is given a sure sense of belonging.

By avoiding the term *mother* to make someone else feel better, I am communicating to a new mother that her accomplishment in safely delivering her baby is nothing special and that even men can have babies and breastfeed, as most national lactation associations now say. It is an attack on women's identities to say that things only women can do are no longer exclusive to women. It is an invasion upon our rightfully earned place in society and a threat to female self-integration to devalue the mother–child dyad relationship. This is a sacred bond, and the words used to describe it should be protected. We deserve to have our spaces respected and honored, not invaded and stolen by men.

WHAT IS A "WOMAN"?

What does it even mean to fit the stereotype of "woman" these days? With no expectation to accept the physiological realities of a female body, the terms *woman, mother, daughter*, and *grandmother* are all arguably up for debate. Our words provide no meaning to serve as guiding principles for young women to emulate and grow into their full identities.

The solution for female happiness and identity Betty Friedan and the second-wave women's movement put forward failed to promote women as unique contributors to society. They failed to protect our roles as mothers and didn't demand accommodation for our needs and goals. Our right to be fully women was lost when we fought for the right to succeed like men. Much of Friedan's inspiration came from an earlier French feminist writer, Simone de Beauvoir.

In 1949 de Beauvoir published her influential book, *The Second Sex*, in which she famously declared "one is not born but becomes a woman," which laid the firm foundation for the gender ideology of what would later become third-wave feminism and is what we are dealing with now.[3] She believed our biology as females had nothing to do with our identities as women, that women were simply nurtured and pushed into female roles, such as motherhood, by culture not nature. It was a dualism that grew upon Descartes' "I think, therefore I am," which ripped the reality of the mind | body integration apart nearly four hundred years earlier. Western culture embraced this dualistic philosophy that said the mind and the body could be separated, and now the very definition of what makes one a woman is up for debate.

De Beauvoir, Friedan, and most recent feminist thinkers have since promoted this idea that we can somehow only find ourselves fully by looking at our external existence and experiences. This belief that we can define and become ourselves by what we do, by what we produce, is a lie that has caused millions of women to relentlessly chase meaning and the right to be seen as human. The truth is that we are human BEINGS, not human DOINGS, and we exist in our fullness right from the moment of our existence. Nothing we do can determine our identities. Identity cannot be created, but only recognized and uncovered. We must first look at ourselves to know our identities as women.

GUIDEPOSTS FOR IDENTITY

"Cogito, ergo sum," René Descartes's famous statement, translated to mean, "I think, therefore I am," has become a fundamental element of Western philosophy. It means that in the face of doubt over one's own existence, one can have certainty, as the very act of thinking connotes being. The primary problem with this thought and the near four hundred years of ensuing philosophy is the presupposition that there already is an "I" in existence who is able to think in the first place. There must be something to have this thought. A brain. A body.

The body, therefore, is the first and primary indicator of the person's existence and their identity, not the mind. Primary traits of identity come from our physical bodies. Our hormones and our natural functions provide outward signs of deeply ingrained truths about who we were created to be. To reject and be in conflict with the primary marker of our unique personal identity leaves one without any sort of anchor to the reality of the human experience.

Secondary identity traits are our preferences. These may not match with the expected gender roles and stereotypes of a given culture, but that does not negate the body, which is always our primary marker of identity. It is when the primary and secondary markers for identities are out of alignment that there are challenges to the gender binary system, which assigns gender roles and expectations based upon biological sex.

The expression of one's unique identity has never been easier than it is today. Strict social stereotypes for identity that once existed have been largely washed away in American culture, and people are free to differentiate and individualize now more than ever. Diversity is valued, and respect for another's personal identity has become the expectation in modern society, which is a wonderful thing.

With the freedom to express identity in an indefinite number of ways, from fashion, to political alignment, to professional choices, it is interesting to note that the crux of the conversation has settled on an individual's personal preferences surrounding their sexuality and gender. It has become normal in the classroom setting for a teacher to ask a student their preferred pronoun along with the pronunciation of their name when they first meet, which is a way to determine the self-identification of one's gender. Interestingly, we don't often hear questions asking someone to tell us how they racially or ethnically identify, nor the age group they identify with.

These things are also tied closely to identity and are observable in our biological makeup. Are these specific identifiers supposed to be assumed based upon observable biological factors, yet hormones and genitals ignored? The idea that one's identity can stretch as far as the imagination can carry is readily accepted and begs the question, what role does nature and biological reality play in identity?

AUTHENTIC IDENTITY

When a society places greater emphasis on the secondary identity traits (such as career choices, preference for sexual partners, fashion expression, choices for recreation), identity representation becomes whatever an individual is currently interested in and attracted to. It can shift and has no deep roots to provide a compass for the human experience. It leaves one totally alone in their individuality, unattached to any other human as it rejects the primary marker of identity as the body. Even the biological relationships are skewed as son, daughter, mother, and father no longer apply when identity shifts so fluidly. We are part of the human family, and our decisions will always affect those around us.

Currently, the accepted idea about identity is that it is not fixed but rather constantly changing and being molded by one's experiences. Life experience certainly plays a role in shaping our preferences and should inform us to make better choices as we grow older. However, if we never accept who we are as human beings, this leaves us perpetually searching and never allows us the freedom of a secure sense of self. If we have no solid sense of self, no character virtues, or core values that we are committed to and work hard to develop, we are not able to grow upon a firm foundation, be at peace with ourselves, or improve continually over time.

We are all students of life, taking in and weighing new information against old. If we are not rooted and continually growing, we can be easily manipulated like leaves blowing wherever new information or circumstance takes us. We will land in places incongruent with our previous sense of self and have no thread to tie our life stories together. Without roots of knowledge anchored deep into our true selves, our identities can shift an innumerable number of times, leaving us feeling less and less sure of who we ever were to begin with.

If instead, we are connected to the basics of our identities provided by the reality of our physical bodies, our DNA, and nature, we are like a strong tree that can bend and sway with the winds. Instead of being blown around or easily influenced, we confidently stand secure because of our established physical reality that keeps us firmly grounded. We are capable of taking in new information without breaking under the pressures of strong personalities or negative social influence. We can sway and move in any direction without losing our roots or sense of self.

KNOWING OUR ROOTS

Our attraction to understanding our roots through DNA speaks volumes about a very natural and normal desire humans have for integrating their heritage into their identities. The DNA industry has grown tremendously in the past decade with groups like 23andMe and Ancestry selling more than twenty-six million at-home DNA test kits.[4] With the results from these massive DNA databases, people are able to connect with genetic relatives and learn more about their genealogical roots. In this instance, we look to our bodies, our chromosomes, to give us clues about who we fully are. We let our bodies reveal to us the hidden secrets they contain and give us a better understanding of ourselves.

Why then do we shun the clues we can observe given by the outward expression of our sex? Are we defining women and men by such strong gender binary stereotypes that we fear accepting the truth our bodies are telling us by the genitalia we were born with? What if the results of our DNA test told us that we were not the nationality that we had believed we were our entire lives? Could we accept that our bodies are telling us the truth of our origins? Or would we cling to a more comfortable identity that made us feel better about ourselves, truthful or not?

Biological ties to family and heritage play a role in identity and self-perception. Even people who are raised far away from their native lands and blood relatives often report feeling a longing for that part of their identities. The connection between people with shared lineage underscores the reality that our bodies have a deep-seated desire for identity and reality that cannot be ignored. When we refuse to accept our bodies, our minds experience dissonance and our spirits grieve the loss of our heritage.

These questions are all at the heart of the identity crisis women are facing today. Our female bodies have become erasable in many ways as we've been taught to ignore the facts as they are being presented to us. We have been encouraged our whole lives to craft identities that match our aspirations and dreams and have not considered whether our primary marker for wholeness is being included.

WHO ARE WE?

We weren't taught to make life choices that considered the total needs of our minds, bodies, or spirits. We weren't told that accepting our bodies first could lead us to knowing ourselves better. We were never advised to consider our years of fertility and the beautiful experience of breastfeeding when we planned our careers. So then, did we allow our bodies to guide us as we grew into women and teach us about our motherhood, or did we stay busy doing all the stuff, never taking time to be who we are?

We weren't taught to take into account the mental energy needed to raise young children, care for a relationship and home, and hold a challenging job simultaneously. We were just expected to somehow know how to successfully balance them all simultaneously. Somehow this juggling act was supposed to make us feel full, and our unique identities were supposed to break free and we would be whole.

We didn't realize that "being busy" isn't the same as being yourself. We don't know ourselves fully because we're simply not paying attention and being mindful of our own needs. Did anyone model for us how to prioritize time for rest and leisure in our schedules, or tell us about the importance of having someone to listen to us and process life's challenges with? Did we learn how to discern our own unique talents and gifts, or were we pushed into a mold for what a fulfilling life was supposed to be?

We aren't given a picture of what living as a whole person looks like, especially as women. Therefore, we do not grow into our full potential of who we were created to be. We begin to believe we've failed when doing all the stuff is hard, when instead we should be questioning whether the stuff is what we were created for. When we struggle, we are led to believe that perhaps our identities are somehow not right, and we look for ways to break free of ourselves, not the unrealistic expectations being placed on us.

Sometimes we escape reality through false personas. With the internet and social media, we can effortlessly create and portray the persona of choice. There is no long-term commitment to a virtual identity, because all that is required is for us to post pictures depicting ourselves the way we want to be perceived. We can publish posts that align with political groups, religious organizations, or social movements online to match our chosen identity, and it requires no real-world action to back up the reality of who we say we are.

We are able to craft complex and intriguing identities that fill our need for acceptance, or even excitement from the comfort of a keyboard while ignoring the fact that these "lives" are fake. These online identities are hollow and ultimately unfulfilling. Yet, our society has moved to celebrating fiction as fact and removing all markers for truth in self-representation.

The attention, praise, and admiration received in these platforms becomes addictive, and we willingly trade the worthy work it takes to make our real lives whole and fulfilling for a cheap and easy substitute that looks and feels good in the moment. But it cannot last, and if the persona presented is false, then the fruits it produces are not real either.

GETTING GROUNDED IN REALITY

Being a mother has been tremendously grounding for me and reminds me of who I am over and over again. I didn't realize that would be the case when I started having children in my early twenties. Having babies was just something I was doing, not who I was; or so I thought. At that point, I shared the same concerns many young mothers have about their education and career goals, wondering if this new baby would somehow prevent me from reaching personal goals and dreams. I was unsure how adding *mother* to my title would change my identity. As I navigated new motherhood as a working mother, I began to realize motherhood is not something that can be compartmentalized. It is not what you're doing; it's who you are. It's who I was always called to be, but I needed to physically have a baby to learn this valuable lesson.

I did worry about finding purpose and success early on, mostly because I had received a secular education that warned me about babies, but these concerns were mostly overridden by my excitement and youthful optimism. I was enthusiastic about starting my new adult life as a married woman and a mother and wanted to embrace my new role. Therefore, I didn't allow myself to focus too much on what I was supposedly giving up as I felt confident that the rewards of family life would far outweigh the challenges. I didn't feel like I was missing out on anything, although it seemed no one was willing to accept that from a twenty-two-year-old mother.

Oftentimes, while I was working on campus, I would encounter people who felt anxious on my behalf. Their concern for me would sometimes leave me unsure of how my decisions would affect my goals and dreams. That environment brought out my insecurities most as I felt eyes and disapproving judgment on me and my baby from students and administrators alike. It seemed those in positions of control and power at the university had clear ideas of what success for their female students looked like, and young motherhood wasn't part of that plan.

One interaction in particular stands out when I think about that time in my life working on campus during my transition into motherhood. I was about eight weeks postpartum after delivering my first child. I had the most beautiful little baby boy who was absolute perfection. He was the kind of baby that people stopped to compliment me on at the mall. Just plain sweet with a big ol' baby head! I was incredibly smitten with him and totally in love.

He had been born the beginning of July during summer break on campus. At the end of August, all the students began moving back into the dorms, and as the leader of our campus ministry program, I would coordinate our student leaders to come and help with move-in days. We'd carry bins and boxes of freshman's stuff up several flights of stairs and welcome the new students to campus with a smile.

Since I had my new baby along with me this year, I stayed near the entrance to the dorms with my baby in a stroller and smiled and welcomed the new students there. One of the top university administrators also came to greet students from this spot. She was an older woman, in her mid-sixties I'd say. I smiled brightly at her and welcomed her to the spot next to me on the sidewalk. I can still remember her polka-dotted hat and wide brimmed sunglasses, which she lowered to look at my son sleeping in his stroller. I fully expected to hear the oohing and aahing that usually went along with seeing my precious baby.

To my surprise, she did not ooh or aah at him. She instead looked me up and down and asked what year student I was. I explained I had graduated over a year ago and now lived and worked on campus with my husband and baby. She shook her head and made a comment about how she hoped I'd be able to use my degree someday since I had gotten a good education.

I was a little bothered by her comment and said that I never thought a degree could be wasted on a mother as they pass on what they've learned to their children. I could tell this deeply annoyed her. She curtly sniped at me, "Well, I'm just so glad I waited to have children until I was much older. So many of my friends are just now waking up to the fact that they wasted the best years of their lives by getting married and having children so young. So much wasted talent."

Wow. That stung. I couldn't believe that woman thought of me as "wasted talent" simply because I had a baby?! I was twenty-three years old with a good marriage, a job I loved, a beautiful healthy baby, and suddenly I would no longer amount to anything in the eyes of this woman? I graduated magna cum laude from her university just a year before, yet I felt like I was already a failure in her eyes. I didn't have anything to say in response, and so I moved slowly away from her, defeated. I was hurt, but something inside me resolved to prove her completely wrong.

SUCCEEDING AS MOTHER

What my husband and I didn't fully appreciate when we chose to be open to children at such a young age was that we were not subscribing to the stereotypical "young professionals" image of having a singular and driven career focus to our lives. Therefore, we were not to be taken seriously or considered professional. We had a broader view of our purpose and saw that children fit with the types of lives we believed would be meaningful and whole.

However, it seemed that we were now considered by many to be reckless, thoughtless, and ill-prepared to meet the demands of the world. Even with college degrees, good jobs, strong work ethics, and a large social support network, we were somehow considered the worst-case scenario to social elites. Young and married with babies. Wasted talent.

The idea that parenthood, motherhood in particular, would ruin our lives was something I refused to accept. I married a man who promised to be my partner and someone who cared about both of our ambitions and passions. He accepted and loved me fully as I am, my mind, my body, and my spirit intact, and swore to help me bring my unique gifts to the world. And I did the same for him.

I knew we would need to be creative and committed to one another's success, but I never believed our children would prevent us from becoming the best versions of ourselves. I suspected they might even hasten the process if we were able to surrender our own timelines and expectations. Now, over a decade and a half into motherhood, I can positively attest that without each of my children I would not be qualified to do the work I am doing today in women's healthcare.

If I had tried to chase a career immediately out of college without making room for my family to grow alongside me, I would have been unqualified for this work. I would have been underdeveloped in the areas that brought me to life, and I may have missed this calling all together. I know this doesn't necessarily apply to all mothers, but personally I would have missed the lessons needed to do what I am now doing well. If I'm going to do anything purposeful on this planet, it will be as a mother because that is who I am and who I was meant to be.

Unfortunately, most young women believe just as that administrator did, that children are a burden too heavy to bear unless you are older, with an established career, and plenty of paid maternity leave from your stable job. I know this isn't true because I have the honor of working with women who defy this antiquated thinking every day, and most of them quite happily.

The truth is that we're not accustomed to accepting women who identify as more than either mothers or employees. We accepted a broken and divided system a long time ago, and now the young women who refuse to acclimate and fit into it are considered "wasted talent." When second-wave feminism placed our careers and roles outside the family on a pedestal, they unwittingly reduced us to worker bees instead of the queen bees we truly are. We willingly accepted that grasping onto one small identifier of ourselves was better than presenting our whole beautiful selves.

I can feel the purpose in my life, and I am energized to get out of bed each day and continue onward. But I know that if I did not have my husband and my children by my side, there would be a huge gap. I feel whole and extremely full doing the work I do because I have not sacrificed any part of myself in the process. I can't do everything all at once, so I've had to take breaks from work for my children, and I've had to take a slower path at times, but that flexibility and surrender has allowed my motherhood to grow and pour out onto others in ways I could have never imagined. All of me is integrated into one cohesive person. Mother, sister, wife, daughter, friend, boss, author, speaker = whole.

THE SPIRIT OF MOTHER

During early motherhood, I learned new truths about my own body and my role in society I could've never imagined before. It was exciting, and I soaked in all the knowledge I could find. I gained so much insight about who I was as a human being, and I experienced a deeper sense of my purpose and identity as my family grew. My little children were teaching me about surrender in totally new ways, and I could tell that as difficult as those lessons were, my spirit was being awakened as I was learning what it meant to live for something greater than myself.

The more I came to identify with and accept my ever-changing hormonal female body, the more concerned I became for women's healthcare and feminism. I began to feel sorry for that women's studies professor, that university administrator, and all the other women in the movement who had settled for the notion that our bodies are inconsequential to our experience on this planet, or worse, that we were victims to our beautiful natural bodies and our babies.

As I thought about everything I had learned about my body and my abilities to succeed in multiple areas of my life in a complete and authentic way, I knew this was what it meant to be a true feminist. I also knew I wasn't the only young woman feeling this way, and my views had nothing to do with a political party or a desire to set women back in the hunt for human equality. Embracing my female mind, body, and spirit made me strong and empowered, not a victim.

I have come to understand that to "mother" is an action and that it is more than a noun that describes who a person is. A mother is a woman who picks others up, oftentimes literally as she's raising babies and toddlers. It is a mother who raises others with care and affection and reminds them they are worthy and valuable at all times. She is the vital ingredient in a society that values one another as she teaches each person to see and care for the needs of others.

I would not have learned the value of my female essence and my predisposition to mother had I not become a physical mother myself. Previously, I placed too much value on masculine traits that tend to be competitive and dominating, but my body literally changed me and taught me to open my eyes to the needs of others.

HEALTHY WOMEN SUPPORT ONE ANOTHER

"Comparison is the thief of joy."

THEODORE ROOSEVELT

What I have learned through my twenties and thirties is many women don't know what it means to be a friend or how to lean on and depend on friends. In our social-media-dependent world, where "friends" refers to the strangers who like our Facebook or Instagram profile, it's difficult to find authentic connection and friendship. Many of us are lonely and searching for our tribes and settle for surface-level connections that require us to be something we're not.

As we lean into and become comfortable expressing our own wholism, we will find opportunities for friendship with women who previously seemed "off limits" because of political, religious, or other social differences. When we find and embrace our unique interests, we're going to find other people who share our passions, and we'll realize that friendship can be found in unlikely places.

Rather than looking for reasons to fight each other, we can erase the lines that have tried to break us down and keep us divided by learning to accept ourselves fully. When we know ourselves and love ourselves the way we were naturally made and gifted, we can drop the insecurity and competitiveness and accept others for their uniqueness as well. We'll see the natural complementarity that exists between all people.

When we reach a state of health where our minds | bodies | spirits are all working cohesively to express the unique people we are, we do not criticize other women. If our feminine nature is alive and well, we know we are called to give encouragement and hope to other people. If we are feeling jealous or judgmental of other women, we need to take a moment and identify the source of that emotion. What untruth about ourselves are we allowing to steal our peace? What trauma is preventing us from celebrating another woman's success?

We need women, healthy and whole, to step forward as mothers to the whole world and set the example for the next generation of what it means to receive and love others. We need to teach our daughters to find their talents and gifts and give them the tools to bring them to the world. We need this next wave of feminism to be focused on wholism so that this upcoming generation of women can bring unity and peace to our world.

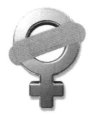

CHAPTER EIGHT

NEXT-GEN FEMINISM

"Strengthen the female mind by enlarging it,
and there will be an end to blind obedience."

MARY WOLLSTONECRAFT,
A VINDICATION OF THE RIGHTS OF WOMAN

As a mother, I often reflect on the world I want my children to grow up in. I think about it for both my sons and daughters. But for my daughters, my heart has a restless concern that the world I am currently raising them in does not recognize their innate dignity as easily as it does their brothers'. My husband and I make conscious and concerted efforts to help our girls see and know their dignity as females, but once they leave the safety of our home, they will be fully subjected to the cultural messages about their value and worth.

I already see it when we're in line at the grocery store and their little eyes wander over the tabloid magazine covers. The natural interest and curiosity sparked by the glamorous women gracing the covers is completely normal, and I can see how their minds are processing the information they receive: beautiful and outgoing equals success and admiration. So, I am not surprised when I walk past my preteen daughter's room and see her looking at herself in the mirror, sucking in her stomach and practicing her pouty lips. As much as we will build her up as parents and tell her how wonderful and unique and special she is, the world is waiting just on the other side of her childhood to toss that all aside and give her marching orders for how she is expected to act and feel about her femaleness.

The best thing I can do as a mother is demonstrate for my children how to search out and find the life that makes me whole. And also, to loudly reject the expectations for me to alter myself, mind, body, or spirit, to fit in. We can all lead the charge and remove the harmful messaging that pits us against our nature and instead create language that encourages each person to find the activities and professions that best depict who they fully are.

FINDING OUR PLACE OF PURPOSE

Each of us has some unique calling or commission we are designed to live out on this earth. It resides deep within our spirits and is unique to us alone, as there is no one else with our gifts, talents, and experiences. It is our unique contribution to humanity, although it may not be something that will be seen by millions or make us famous; perhaps only very few people will witness our genius at work. It may not even be something that we do but could be something our presence pulls out in others. Maybe our very presence in the world makes other people better. What a gift that type of spirit is to others. When we are living in accord with our purpose, we experience integration and wholeness. An important part of creating a new wave of the women's movement is that we acknowledge each person's unique calling. Women are not going to fit neatly into any one place because, while we are similar in our biology, our temperaments and talents differ tremendously.

Our activism needs to support women wherever and however they are called to act. Author, radio show host, and comedian Jennifer Fulwiler talks about the desire each person has to uncover and live the unique purpose of their lives. She calls that thing that burns hot and bright deeply within us a blue flame. It is something that gets us excited about life and makes us a little scared to actually do it. In her book *Your Blue Flame: Drop the Guilt and Do What Makes You Come Alive,* she says a blue flame has three elements:

1. We were meant to do it.
2. It fills us with energy.
3. It benefits others.[1]

We each have a blue flame. We have something that we've been preparing to say or do our entire lives. The scary thing to realize and understand is that if we don't discover and do this thing, then it will never get done because we are the only one who can contribute this thing to the world. Doing this thing is part of our very identities, and when we embrace it, the world will be better.

Finding it and grabbing on to it will allow you to live fully on fire as the amazing woman we were created to be. But we can't find it unless we know and accept ourselves first. When we know and accept our whole unique identities, minds, bodies, and spirits, we can observe the places where we come most fully alive and what causes our creative capacities to pour out of us for the benefit of ourselves and others. We must each learn to be uniquely ourselves as we set the example for the next generation of women and give them the courage to dream outside the confines of societal expectation.

MY BLUE FLAME

We can't assume that all women will have the same blue flames as one another; housekeeping certainly is NOT my passion, although I have friends who love putting things in order. It's taken me a long time to accept that it's okay and that I'm not a failure as a wife and mother because I have approximately a dozen loads of unwashed clothes sitting by my washing machine at all times. We're simply wired differently, and I have my own gifts that bring light and order into the world. I have found that community activism, working with women, and encouraging others through teaching, speaking, and writing really bring me to life. I have unique experiences and a voice that can effect change for other women, and when I use it, I come alive. It's as if I were meant to do this exact thing.

When I am speaking and writing about the future of feminism and the beauty of women's bodies, I feel right. My blue flame is lit, and my creative spark is lit up. I feel it when I work with women learning to breastfeed. When I see the work happening each day in Guiding Star centers (the women's health and medical centers that my nonprofit opens) and the lives being changed because of the vision I have for women's healthcare, it sometimes overwhelms me with a deep gratitude for the call I've been given. I feel whole.

As I've been writing this book, I've had moments when I've sat in stunned silence recognizing that every part of my life has in fact prepared me to do this. I have been equipped in countless ways to promote a social movement toward wholism through the delivery of women's healthcare. This work is authentic to me and my experiences because it comes from the life I have lived. From my childhood growing up surrounded by nature on a dairy farm, to my early years of motherhood spent on a university campus, to my education and diverse friendships, to founding a nonprofit, to my unique gifts and strengths, to now being the mother of a large family; I am meant to contribute my voice and worldview to the world through wholistic feminism. It energizes me, and I believe the work I'm doing will benefit others.

We each have something like this deep within us. The key is for us to broaden our horizons and shake off the expectations and pressures women currently feel so that we can be whole and find our unique voices, which speak to our authentic identities and purposes. If we blindly continue to walk the expected pathways for women, we risk living out the purpose of our lives.

SILENCING THE CRITICS AND GENDER STEREOTYPES

Jennifer Fulwiler writes comedically about her personal experience of finding and embracing her blue flame. She bravely stepped far outside the norm for a suburban wife and mother of six young children when she decided to write, produce, and take her own stand-up comedy act on the road across the United States, with her children in tow. The decision seemed crazy to most people, and she faced a lot of cautionary comments from others indicating their opinion that this might be a terrible idea. In her book she says,

> "What I am is a person who has battled through guilt and fear and other people's opinions about how I should be living and came out the other side with a life that I love." [2]
>
> JENNIFER FULWILER

There is no shortage of opinions about what is the right thing for women, especially mothers to do with their lives. Many of us have been told very directly what and when it is acceptable for us to chase our dreams. Many of us feel immense pressure to think and act in accord with an ideology that is safe. The wildest and most beautiful thing we can do with our lives is to become exactly who we were created to be: fully ourselves, unsuppressed, whole!

It might feel really uncomfortable as we address our own deep-seated ideas about what are appropriate roles for men or women. We may have grown up with traditional gender roles and can't imagine how society would look with men and women doing the things that really bring them to life. I challenge you to trust that when each person is healthy, whole, and in line with their own nature, that society and culture will come alive in ways that will inspire greatness, goodness, truth, and beauty. Humanity was made for greatness; let's allow it to happen!

WHERE DO WOMEN BELONG?

Okay, but practically speaking, how do we answer that age-old question that has been plaguing women since the onset of the feminist movement: to work or not to work? Since women are so good at relationships and caring for others, and the very essence of our femininity is to "mother," shouldn't women who have children then stay at home and care for the family?

The topic of working mothers has been a hot-button issue in online forms and women's groups for many years, with an uptick in the past few years. Many young women whose mothers chose to pursue careers full-time are now facing motherhood themselves and are struggling to come to terms with their own childhoods and the effects of their mother's work on them. While other young women, like me, whose mothers did stay home throughout their childhood, are wondering how to find fulfillment and reach their own definitions of success while also raising children.

We all have the same fears; are we bad moms for choosing to work, or underachievers for choosing to not work? Are we simply repeating patterns of male domination with our decision? At the end of our lives, will we be satisfied or confident in our decision? Is there a right answer to whether or not women belong in the home or the workplace?

There is not an easy one-size-fits-all answer to these questions. The bottom line is that our world is hurting tremendously because of a lack of women's understanding and acceptance of our feminine gifts and of our abilities to recognize and nurture the others around them. We women have not been raised to know ourselves fully and are under-informed about how to bring our blue flames to the world. When we do not know or embrace our essence as life-bearers and bestowers of dignity upon the vulnerable, the world has lost our most valuable contribution—the concept of what it means to truly embrace, welcome, and mother another.

OUTSIDE THE HOME

The home is certainly not the only place where mothers are needed. When we look at the problems facing many school systems, you can't help but feel that these hurting children need to be surrounded and loved by mothers. It's clear they need someone to be their cheerleader and sit alongside them as they work through challenges, celebrating their successes.

When we look at the almost slave-like conditions of many corporate American office buildings, where people work upwards of eighty hours a week without so much as a pat on the back or uplifting eye contact, does it make you wonder how much more satisfying their lives would be if there was someone in their office who recognized and applauded their efforts?

The question should not be whether or not women belong at home or out in the world; the question should be how could the world survive if women stay exclusively in the home? We need the gifts and contributions of women to personalize and give value to others around them. Some women will feel a strong call toward a certain profession, and for the sake of that field, they absolutely should pursue their talents and passions. Women must pursue their blue flames wherever they call, but they must do so as women, as mothers.

REDEFINING SUCCESS

If a woman is to climb the corporate ladder and become the highest member of an organization, yet she is a ruthless and self-seeking individual, it does no good for the women's movement. In fact, it harms our efforts to say women are capable of succeeding when an aggressive, power-hungry woman meets the male definition of success. No, what we need are women to rise to the highest ranks with all the qualities of motherhood and femininity intact.

Imagine a CEO of a Fortune 500 company who is focused on the individual employee's well-being? Wouldn't it catch the attention of the world if she remembered her staff's birthdays?! I can just see the headlines: "CEO Frosts Birthday Cupcakes, Losing Her Edge?" Currently, it's assumed that any breakthrough of feminine qualities in the workplace is a failure of leadership. The Sheryl Sandbergs of the world have done a tremendous job of bringing their motherhood to the workplace and making room for mothers to rise, yet they must walk a careful line to not be seen as too feminine, lest they destroy their professional reputation.

Women in the workplace who recognize the individual dignity of everyone else in the office are a radical testimony to the role and need of women in society. They can remind the world that every person matters and that they deserve to be treated with dignity, no matter their position. That is the type of change women can bring to our culture when they choose to use their gifts and talents outside the home.

When more women have moved into leadership roles across all spheres of society, including business, politics, and religion, we will see the contributions of those who mother, no matter if it is in the home or in the office, as a vital part of our cultural health. Mothers will no longer fear being penalized for taking a leave from work to stay home with their child for a period of time. It will be seen as valuable investment in future generations. Women will no longer feel the need to assert a masculine framework to define their success. The world will begin to understand and see that the psychological health and well-being of employees and students are improved the more the feminine qualities are encouraged and embraced in the world.

Success for all women should be the measure to which she is able to become the fullest version of her unique self and bring those qualities to the world. Women should be universally admired for the impact they have upon others and the love and compassion they draw out and multiply around them. Success should have much less to do with accolades and status, and much more to do with relationships and impact.

AT HOME, RAISING BABIES

Women in the home are just as necessary to infuse the youngest members of our society with their own sense of dignity and value. Parents, both women and men, are the first people who communicate to a child their right to be treated well and to be recognized as an equal human person in our society. A culture of justice and equality is built upon these core ideas. When considering who is best equipped to share this message with the youngest and most impressionable in our society, we must look at the gifts of both men and women and consider the needs of young children and their abilities to receive these messages. We cannot abandon the obvious truth of biological reality when considering what is best for a child.

When we become parents, we must put aside our own desires in deference for the well-being of our dependent child; both as mothers and as fathers, we must care about the needs of the new child in our family first. The reality of our female bodies is that we are capable of conceiving, sustaining, birthing, and nurturing a child for a number of years. This cannot be erased as a biological fact, as it is important for both the mother and the child's identity in relationship to one another. Mothers thrive when they are given the praise they deserve for bringing new life into the world. Children thrive when their mothers recognize their legitimate needs and give them the attention and nourishment their bodies and minds deserve.

We are not interchangeable as mothers and fathers when it comes to the physical aspects of caring for babies. Our female bodies give us a pretty good guide for staying close to our babies throughout the first two years of life as they breastfeed and form strong attachments and self-assurance. If we are away from our babies for too long in the early months, our leaking breasts will quickly remind us that there is a little person that needs us. There is nothing better for our babies than to have their mothers available and close to them. This could be accomplished by staying home with them, or by corporations and workplaces creating policies and spaces that welcome children to be close to their parents at work. However it is accomplished, we need to recognize the truth that women's bodies are telling society that mothers and babies need one another.

It is our jobs as mothers and fathers to look objectively at our children and to understand their needs. Then we must take the actions necessary to meet their needs so that they grow up knowing they are worthy of being treated with dignity and respect. The next generation of feminism needs to understand the human need for relationship and human bonds.

LOVING OUR FEMALE BODIES AND DEFENDING THE WORK THEY DO

The truth is our female bodies are always at work wherever they are, in the workplace or at home. They have the most important work of all to do. Female bodies have never been the real problem. Our fertility, childbearing, and breastfeeding abilities are not liabilities; they are essential contributions to the health and continuation of our species. Let's say it again, a little louder for the people in the back: **Our bodies are NOT the problem, a society that doesn't understand or accept them IS**.

We need to reject the premise that there is something wrong with how women's bodies work, as that makes altering our bodies an acceptable solution to challenges. Our daughters' feminism will boldly state that if our fertility, childbearing, and breastfeeding is creating a difficulty for our employers or schools, then we all need to rethink how we are doing things because we are not the ones who should be expected to change. Society needs to adjust its ideas about what is an acceptable way for women to be present in it.

We need to change the narrative that says women are only allowed to be present in a certain way. The norm should never be an altered and artificial female body. That is unfair to our daughters and robs them of the primary guideposts for understanding their full identities. They can't know themselves if they don't even know their own bodies.

I have met far too many young women in unexpected pregnancies who seemed genuinely shocked by their situation. These girls were either not aware of the reality of their natural abilities or health, or were led to believe that condoms and contraceptives could perfectly circumvent the laws of nature. Young girls must be guided into their newly fertile and young adult bodies. They need to understand the reality of what their female bodies are capable of. The onset of menstruation or the ability to conceive should never come as a surprise.

If the younger generation is not mentored and prepared for the reality of their bodies, then they will be inclined to shun their womanhood. Girls who work tirelessly to have sculpted abs, or who out of disdain for their feminine curves develop eating disorders to appear perpetually preadolescent, are grasping for an altered and unnatural "normal," having nothing to do with the biological reality of a woman's body. Instead, it is a vain attempt to participate in a predominantly male-normed society. It is a destruction of women's natural rhythms and abilities, without any appreciation for the beauty they are capable of creating, and it is not healthy.

If a young girl apathetically believes that sexual activity doesn't naturally lead to pregnancy, or feels like a pregnancy is not "normal," she has passively accepted the male-normative worldview and expectation for health. Our young women should never be surprised by how their bodies work, nor feel ashamed of their functions. They should see successful women on the covers of magazines who are living fully alive in their female bodies.

LEADING BY EXAMPLE

In 2017, Australian Senator Larissa Waters made history after she became the first mother to breastfeed her baby openly in Australia's Parliament. Her baby, Alia, became a regular attendee at Australia's Senate and made history as her mother addressed the chamber while nursing her at three months old. Far from being discouraged, Waters felt supported by her fellow senators' warm smiles. But this change came relatively recently as reported in an article by the *Telegraph* newspaper:

> "Previously, mothers had to leave the chamber to breastfeed and were required to seek a proxy for any votes. The Senate—at Ms. Waters' urging—has also changed its rules to ensure mothers or fathers can enter the Senate to briefly assist with the care of children. I am so proud that my daughter Alia is the first baby to be breastfed in the Federal Parliament," Ms. Waters said in May. "We need more women and parents in Parliament. And we need more family-friendly and flexible workplaces, and affordable childcare, for everyone."[3]

Our daughters' feminism will recognize that mothers like Ms. Waters are not the unique exception to women. There are millions of mothers who desire to continue using their intellect and talents after having children. With some creativity and policy changes, such as flexible work arrangements and easier to access childcare, their voices can continue to be heard.

Here in the United States, we are seeing a confusing message from our legislators with regards to their understanding and acceptance of the needs of mothers. While mothers are encouraged to breastfeed and there have been major wins with the establishment of lactation rooms on the Capitol Hill complex, [4] a code of conduct change took place in early 2021 in the US House of Representatives.

Led by House Speaker Nancy Pelosi the House removed gendered language and replaced them with gender-inclusive terms in its official language. Terms for familial relationships, such as mother, father, daughter, son, sister, and brother, have been swapped with terms such as parent, child, and sibling.[5] Again, while this change may seem small and inconsequential to some, it will irrevocably shift the dynamic of the groups of women who have found sisterhood and relationship with one another over their shared experience of working and pumping at Capitol Hill.

> "Ellen Nedrow, the scheduler for Sen. Jay Rockefeller, D-W.Va., started the Congressional Nursing Moms group in 2013, after talking with another mother while waiting to pump.
>
> "We wanted a place to ask questions, share advice and talk. I decided to stop wishing it already existed and put up a sign about our first meeting," Nedrow said.
>
> The Nursing Moms group has an email list and meets for monthly lunches in the Capitol. Discussions revolve around nursing questions and "typical parenting topics like birthday parties, traveling with small children, recipes and of course sleep; [as well as] concerns that we all share as staffers, such as long days and late votes," Nedrow said."[6]

What was once a point of nonpolitical community and bipartisan agreement has now become politically contentious and limiting. It is unnecessary and unwise to remove these titles for women because we lose feminine privilege when we lose feminine words to protect them.

THE IDEAL WORKPLACE

I spoke about my belief that women are desperately needed in the world, but we are currently telling our daughters they are expected to compartmentalize their career and families into two separate boxes that should not be opened at the same time. Women are expected to be either good employees or good mothers. One or the other, not both. Lactation rooms are a wonderful acknowledgment of the ways that we contribute beyond our jobs, but they are merely a polite nod that many employers hope will pacify and distract us from the other major flaws in their views of motherhood.

Take for example the employee policies at major companies such as Facebook, Google, and Apple that cover the cost for egg freezing for their female employees.[7] Young women are encouraged to freeze their eggs so that they can put off having children during their years of optimal fertility. However, there is no employee benefit for childcare stipends or on-site childcare facilities.

What are we saying to young women when we tell them there is no accommodation for their children, but that we're willing to pay thousands of dollars to chemically alter their fertility to invasively extract their eggs and freeze them for later use? As a society, we are saying women are most valuable as childless employees, that motherhood is something they should put off (perhaps indefinitely?) and that women should give all their time and attention to their jobs and career advancements. When delaying and avoiding motherhood is incentivized, we are saying that women are most valuable to society when they are not mothers.

Think about how this idea about women's usefulness and value affects young girls. We are raising our girls in a culture that says our productivity as an employee or worker is what gives us value to the outside world. We are measuring our "success" by a standard that has been set up for men to be most successful. Men who are free from the biological blessings of childbearing can easily outpace women who are in the caregiving role in terms of being singularly focused on accomplishing tasks, but are they missing the bigger picture?

An important piece is missing in large corporations and businesses that do not include the voices of caregivers, mothers in particular. We need the people who remind big companies that people should always be put first, before profit, and if a profit comes at the expense of human dignity, that it is hurtful for our world. Some of the people who might be less "productive" to a company's bottom line are the most critical people for them to employ if they want to contribute to a healthy world. What if we rejected this idea that productivity is the way to measure "success" and instead considered that it is just as important to be truly present to others?

How do we attract these women into companies and optimize their success? Flexible work hours, benefits for families that can include healthcare and childcare perks, sick time for parents to be with children who need them, and options for remote work. Being good bosses should look less like demanding control over time and setting strict expectations for how and where work is completed, and instead being clear about the expectations for a position and working with an employee to see how they can effectively achieve those goals. When mothers are given the ability to take care of what truly matters most in their lives, their children and families, they will be free to focus on the work at hand without anxiety.

Investment in other people is no less valuable, and perhaps should even be argued is MORE valuable than investing in products. The return on investment that our daughters' feminism will bring is, in culture, being changed through authentic relationships that communicate the value of all people. Our daughters' feminism will say that it is just as successful to build strong communities and relationships as it is to build structures and produce products for sale.

A NEW FEMINIST DECLARATION

For our daughters' sakes, let us give them the ability to begin afresh with a new movement that can represent and unite all women together in goodwill. Let's give them the words that release them from victimhood by instilling a confidence and self-assurance of their dignity and worth.

Just as the first feminists began with a Declaration of Sentiments at Seneca Falls, let's begin this new era of the women's movement with a new declaration. A Declaration of Inalienable Truths that outline the worth and value of the female contributions. A declaration that proudly asserts the natural abilities of women's bodies and declares them to be faultless in the struggles of the human condition.

Let's do something amazing for our daughters and give them a framework to grow upon that places them in the position of strength and presupposes their equality with men. Let's assume the best of men's willingness to come alongside as partners on the quest for true equality in all ways; men typically rise to the standard we women set. Let's build a movement that reminds our daughters they do not have to sacrifice and divide themselves up to build a future, but they are most valuable in their whole. That ALL of them matters. Let's build a new and Wholistic Feminism.

A NEW DECLARATION
ON BEHALF OF ALL WOMEN

THE TRUTHS OF WOMANHOOD

When, in the course of human events, it becomes necessary for a portion of the human family to assert their God-given dignity and respect due to them, it is important that they make clear the desired solutions to injustice moving forward. It is also important that the establishment of their God-given rights and abilities be enshrined as self-evident and inalienable truths for all of humanity to ponder, embrace, and pass on to subsequent generations.

We hold these truths to be self-evident: that all men and women are created equal, yet uniquely different in their natural abilities and talents; that men and women can live and work harmoniously together; and that each brings valuable insights to society through their biological differences.

All humans are endowed by their Creator with certain inalienable rights and natural abilities; that among these rights are life, liberty, and the pursuit of happiness; and among their natural inalienable abilities are their bodily functions of fertility and procreation.

To secure these rights governments are instituted, deriving their powers from the consent of the governed. Whenever any form of government becomes destructive of these rights and abilities, it is the right of those who suffer from it to insist upon the institution of laws and policies of protection, laying its foundation on such principles of respect for the nature of humanity, and organizing its powers in such form, as to them shall seem most likely to affect their safety and happiness.

As representatives of all human females, in the many vast and diverse circumstances of existence, we endeavor to create a better situation for all of our daughters. To create the conditions that will protect the undeniable value and worth of all women, we move away from sentimentality and embrace the objective similarities that all women experience with their female bodies.

Therefore, we seek a world that will celebrate the birth of a female child and declare their equal position and worth with all male children;

Where equal opportunities for education for all children is standard, as this is the tool for which all humans endeavor to improve their station and situation in society. And that in our educational institutions, girls be included in all areas of study, for the ability to learn all topics is not a point of gender difference;

That all children be allowed the freedom of self-expression of their unique personalities, and that strict cultural expectations for male and female roles not pertaining to the natural biological realities of their bodies be avoided;

That both girls and boys be welcomed into a wide variety of hobbies, sports, and careers, as befitting their unique talents and abilities;

That organizations, clubs, and religious institutions that recognize and ennoble the sexual difference of females and males in such a way as to elevate both of the sexes to a position of equal esteem and honor be respected in their rights to include only one of the sexes as participants, and that spaces intended for only one of the sexes to exist in be preserved for the comfort and companionship of the sex they serve;

That education on the biological reality for the healthy female and male body be given to all children so that a love and understanding of who they are can grow;

That respect for children's natural innocence and naivete be observed in their education on biological sexual difference and that adult intrusion and encroachment be avoided as children navigate their developing bodies and emotions free of scandal;

That boys and girls be taught to understand the biological and emotional differences between the sexes so as to better respect the needs of the opposite sex;

That the expectation for all boys and girls concerning sexual acts be of full consent and that violence, aggression, or manipulation be avoided at all costs;

That boys and men be educated on the changing fertile cycle of women so as to be accountable to an expectation of cooperation with her in family planning and sexual activity;

That all girls be told that being fertile and the ability to ovulate is a gift that should be carefully protected and preserved;

That menstruation not be met with shame or secrecy, but rather that we celebrate the onset of fertility and womanhood and remove the stigma of a natural healthy function of the female body;

That every pregnancy, whether planned or unplanned, be seen as a tremendous accomplishment for a woman's body, and that the growing child be viewed as a gift to society;

Where our medical institutions and medical providers view the natural female body as a healthy and intact system and not accept the alteration, suppression, or destruction of the reproductive functions as healthy or acceptable care;

Where pregnant women be given excellent healthcare, including emotional and physical support, and also a voice in their choices about labor and delivery and that medical providers work with them to assure safe delivery of their babies;

Where women are welcomed into the workforce as mothers and that employers creatively ease the challenges of family life through maternity/paternity leave policies, childcare stipends or on-site care, and spaces and break times to attend to pumping breastmilk or the other needs of their children;

That girls understand that they are free to be whoever they uniquely are, expressing their gifts and talents in whatever arena they are called to. We long to see women represented in all areas of society so as to bring the uniquely feminine perspective to all areas of commerce, community, and culture.

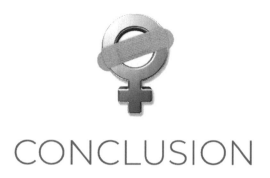

CONCLUSION

The feminine body is beautiful, powerful, and sacred. Looking at women's bodies, we are aware of our biological realities—what makes us different from men, what makes us powerful in our unique way. These natural feminine characteristics and abilities are the commonality that should bring together all women. When we come together as mothers, exercising in a mama and baby class, breastfeeding in public, or simply meeting at the park where our children play together, we are finding our commonality.

What is at stake by continuing to ignore the sacred bond of our feminine essence, and the connectivity that should exist between all human beings, is a world that continues to grow more divided by the day. Without women understanding and knowing our vital contribution to culture, there will be no peace. We are meant to be whole, connected and dependent upon one another for our health and wellbeing. We are the mothers, bestowers of dignity, and the peacekeepers.

As a society, we must do better for women. We need to provide better education to our young girls and boys, to prepare them for what is ahead for them, what their bodies are capable of, and how to understand fertility. If there is understanding, then everyone can take responsibility for their actions.

We must know and remember our bodies are naturally good, and we are made to be in relationship with others. If we all focus on our goodness, there will be no need to dwell on weaknesses. We will only see inherent beauty and power in others and ourselves.

Let us advocate for better policies to allow women to participate in the world without the expectation that they somehow suppress their femininity in order to fit in and perform to male expectations.

Let us advocate for better healthcare for women that understands and embraces women's natural bodies without suppressing them. We need to trust that women's bodies are healthiest in their natural state.

Together, let's support women in their dreams, their ambitions, and their struggles. If we can create a society and a culture where it is safe to be wholly female or wholly male, we will be able to see the world come alive with creativity, love, and acceptance. What a world that will be.

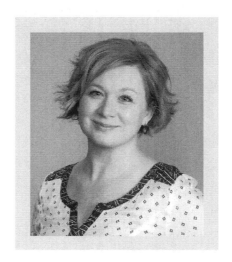

ABOUT THE AUTHOR

Leah A. Jacobson MA, IBCLC, resides in small-town central Minnesota with her husband, Josh, and their seven children. She has been working with young people and mothers since 2000. Amidst growing her family, she received her master's degree in health and wellness, with a special focus on women's health and lactation care and became an international board-certified lactation consultant.

Leah founded The Guiding Star Project, a 501c3 non-profit organization, in 2011 after feeling called to help women and families by providing resources that honor natural law and promote wholistic feminism. Leah sees her work with Guiding Star as a proactive approach to addressing root causes of cultural inequalities facing women in healthcare and bodily autonomy. Her hope is that Guiding Star centers will open across the United States and serve as beacons of hope, joy, and truth—safe havens upholding human dignity at all stages of life.

www.leahajacobson.com

GUIDING STAR

Leah A. Jacobson, MA, IBCLC, has been working professionally with young women and new mothers for over a decade. In hundreds of interactions with women, she came to see and understand the fear, loneliness, and confusion many modern women are experiencing with embracing their role as mothers. Her work led her to found a nonprofit organization in 2012, The Guiding Star Project, which is focused on opening up comprehensive women's healthcare centers across the nation.

These centers spread a narrative framework for natural and affirming healthcare for women's unique bodies. In her first book, *Wholistic Feminism*, Leah lays out the affirming worldview that women's bodies are not broken and that modern medical practices that alter, suppress, or destroy women's naturally healthy and fertile bodies are the antithesis of true women's liberation. With a look back at the successes and failures of the women's movement, Leah paints a hopeful picture of what the future of feminism will look like in America.

www.guidingstarproject.com

CONNECT WITH LEAH

Leah teaches a variety of online courses and is available for speaking engagements. To inquire about availability, email her team at: leah@wholisticfeminism.com

ADDITIONAL RESOURCES

To find a Guiding Star Center near you:

guidingstarproject.com/our-affiliates

Natural Fertility

FACTS – https://factsaboutfertility.org

Natural Womanhood – https://naturalwomanhood.org

FertilityCare – https://fertilitycare.org

FEMM – https://femmhealth.org

SymptoPro – https://symptopro.org

Billings – https://boma-usa.org

Family of the Americas – https://familyplanning.net

Marquette – https://vitaefertility.com

Couple to Couple League – https://ccli.org

Creighton Model – https://creightonmodel.com

Managing Your Fertility – https://managingyourfertility.com

Natural Childbirth

Bradley Method – http://bradleybirth.com

Evidence Based Birth – https://evidencebasedbirth.com

Spinning Babies – https://spinningbabies.com

Lamaze – https://lamaze.org

Birthing from Within – https://birthingfromwithin.com

Midwifery Model of Care – https://mana.org/about-midwives/midwifery-model

Ina May Gaskin and The Farm – http://thefarmmidwives.org

VBAC Facts – https://vbacfacts.com

Improving Birth Coalition – http://motherfriendly.org

Hypnobirthing – https://us.hypnobirthing.com

Breastfeeding Support

ILCA – https://ilca.org

USLCA – https://uslca.org

La Leche League International – https://llli.org

Baby Cafe – https://babycafeusa.org

Breastfeeding USA – https://breastfeedingusa.org

Kelly Mom – https://kellymom.com

Birth Trauma

Solace for Mothers – http://.solaceformothers.org

Infertility/Miscarriage/Infant Loss

NaPro Technology – https://naprotechnology.com

Share Pregnancy and Infant Loss Support – https://nationalshare.org

Mary Haseltine – https://maryhaseltine.com/p/pregnancy-loss.html

Hannah's Tears – https://hannahstears.org

Filumena Birth and Bereavement - https://filumenabirth.com

Postpartum Support

Postpartum Support International - https://postpartum.net

ENDNOTES

CHAPTER ONE

1. Our History. (n.d.). EMILY's List. Retrieved November 11, 2018, from https://www.emilyslist.org/pages/entry/our-history

2. Swanson, E. (2017, December 7). *Poll: Few Identify as Feminists, But Most Believe in Equality of Sexes*. HuffPost. https://www.huffpost.com/entry/feminism-poll_n_3094917?fb_comment_id=182860378531192_4098989124940 03#f2470b0bd

3. Editors of Merriam-Webster. (2020, November 29). *Why Merriam-Webster Chose "Feminism" for 2017 Word of the Year*. The Merriam-Webster.Com Dictionary. https://www.merriam-webster.com/words-at-play/woty2017-top-looked-up-words-feminism

4. *Definition of Feminism*. (n.d.). Merriam Webster Online Dictionary. Retrieved December 11, 2017, from https://www.merriam-webster.com/dictionary/feminism?src=search-dict-hed

5. *Declaration of Sentiments - Women's Rights National Historical Park* (US National Park Service). (1848, July). National Park Service. https://www.nps.gov/wori/learn/historyculture/declaration-of-sentiments.htm

6. Betty Friedan, *The Feminine Mystique*. New York: W.W. Norton & Company, 1963. 422.

7. Brown, H. G. (1962). *Sex and the Single Girl.* Bernard Geis Associates.

CHAPTER TWO

1. Menand, L. (2021, February 3). *Betty Friedan and Books as Bombs.* The New Yorker. https://www.newyorker.com/magazine/2011/01/24/books-as-bombs

2. Betty Friedan, *The Feminine Mystique.* New York: W.W. Norton & Company, 1963.

3. Betty Friedan, *The Feminine Mystique.* New York: W.W. Norton & Company, 1963. Pg. 422.

4. Women in the Workforce—United States: Quick Take. (2020, October 14). *Catalyst.* https://www.catalyst.org/research/women-in-the-workforce-united-states/. (Accessed December 2020).

5. Bureau of Labor Statistics, "Table 11: Employed Persons by Detailed Occupation, Sex, Race, and Hispanic or Latino Ethnicity," *Current Population Survey* (2020). (Accessed December 2020)

6. Menand, L. (2021, February 3). *Betty Friedan and Books as Bombs.* The New Yorker. https://www.newyorker.com/magazine/2011/01/24/books-as-bombs

7. Ekeocha, O. (2012, August) An African Woman's Open Letter to Melinda Gates. *Pontifical Council for the Laity.* http://www.laici.va/content/laici/en/sezioni/donna/notizie/an-african-woman-s-open-letter-to-melinda-gates.html (Accessed November 2020)

8. CheckYourPriviledge.com, no longer published.

9. Digest of Education Statistics. (n.d.). *Historical summary of faculty, enrollment, degrees conferred, and finances in degree-granting postsecondary institutions: Selected years, 1869-70 through 2015-16.*

National Center for Education Statistics. Retrieved January 1, 2021, from https://nces.ed.gov/programs/digest/d17/tables/dt17_301.20.asp

10. DuBois, Ellen Carol; Dumenil, Lynn (2009). Through Women's Eyes: An American History with Documents (2nd ed. ed.). Boston: Bedford/St. Martin's. p. 690.

11. Stritof, S. (2019, December 1). *Estimated Median Age of First Marriage by Gender: 1890 to 2018.* The Spruce. https://www.thespruce.com/estimated-median-age-marriage-2303878

12. Ortiz-Ospina, E., & Roser, M. (2019, November 1). *In most countries the gender pay gap has decreased in the last couple of decades.* Our World in Data. https://ourworldindata.org/economic-inequality-by-gender#in-most-countries-the-gender-pay-gap-has-decreased-in-the-last-couple-of-decades

13. Calhoun, A. (2017, October). *The New Midlife Crisis for Women.* Oprah.Com. https://www.oprah.com/sp/new-midlife-crisis.html Accessed November 2017

14. Stevenson, Betsey & Wolfers, Justin. (2009). *The Paradox of Declining Female Happiness.* Federal Reserve Bank of San Francisco, Working Paper Series. 1.000-48.000. 10.24148/wp2009-11.

15. Carey, B., & Gebeloff, R. (2018, April 7). *Many People Taking Antidepressants Discover They Cannot Quit.* The New York Times. https://www.nytimes.com/2018/04/07/health/antidepressants-withdrawal-prozac-cymbalta.html

16. Coaston, J. (2019, May 28). *Intersectionality, explained: meet Kimberlé Crenshaw, who coined the term.* Vox. https://www.vox.com/the-highlight/2019/5/20/18542843/intersectionality-conservatism-law-race-gender-discrimination

17. Berry, M., & Chenoweth, E. (n.d.). *Who Made the Women's March?* Square Space. Retrieved March 10, 2021, from https://static1.squarespace.com/static/5161b65fe4b0c98010aa8cd7/t/5cf838c935b8040001f2ff03/1559771339751/Berry+and+Chenoweth_Women%27s+March_2018.pdf

18. Carney, E. N. (2017, January 19). *Who's Behind the Women's March?* The American Prospect. https://prospect.org/power/behind-women-s-march/

19. *Feminism.* (n.d.). Merriam Webster Online Dictionary. Retrieved January 1, 2018, from https://www.merriam-webster.com/words-at-play/woty2017-top-looked-up-words-feminism#:~:text=Feminism%20was%20first%20entered%20in,of%20women's%20rights%20and%20interests.%E2%80%9D

20. Alice Von Hildebrand

21. Guidos, Rhina (January 21, 2017). "Though snubbed by Women's March, pro-life groups will still participate". *Catholic News.*

CHAPTER THREE

1. Wilcox, A. J., Dunson, D., & Baird, D. D. (2000). The timing of the "fertile window" in the menstrual cycle: day specific estimates from a prospective study. *BMJ (Clinical research ed.), 321*(7271), 1259–1262. https://doi.org/10.1136/bmj.321.7271.1259

2. "The Discovery of Different Types of Cervical Mucus and the Billings Ovulation Method", Professor Erik Odeblad, Bulletin of the Natural Family Council of Victoria, ISSN 0321-7567, Vol 21 No 3 September 1994, pp3-35.

3. *NaPro Technology Infertility.* (n.d.). NaPro Technology. Retrieved March 3, 2021, from https://naprotechnology.com/infertility/

4. *NaProTECHNOLOGY vs. IVF.* (n.d.). FertilityCareTM Services of Venice. Retrieved March 11, 2021, from http://www.fertilitycarevenice.org/naprotechnology-vs-ivf

5. Postpartum Support International. (2020, December 11). *Postpartum Post-Traumatic Stress Disorder | Postpartum Support International (PSI).* Postpartum Support International— PSI. https://www.postpartum.net/learn-more/postpartum-post-traumatic-stress-disorder/#:%7E:text=Approximately%20 9%25%20of%20women%20experience,Prolapsed%20cord

6. Dekker, R. (2020, June 29). *Evidence on: Birthing Positions.* Evidence Based Birth®. https://evidencebasedbirth.com/evidence-birthing-positions/

7. Harper, B., & Arms, S. (2005). *Gentle Birth Choices* (New Edition of Gentle Birth Choices Boxed Set ed.). Healing Arts Press. Pg. 217

8. *Brought to Bed: Childbearing in America 1750 to 1950* (Paperback) by Judith Walzer Leavitt [1988 Edition]. (1679). Judith Walzer Leavitt.

9. *Jimmy Carter National Historic Site—Presidents: A Discover Our Shared Heritage Travel Itinerary.* (n.d.). National Park Service. Retrieved September 19, 2020, from https://www.nps.gov/nr/travel/presidents/jimmy_carter_nhs.html

10. Pollesch, J. (2018, May 16). *Twilight Sleep | The Embryo Project Encyclopedia.* The Embryo Project Encyclopedia. https://embryo.asu.edu/pages/twilight-sleep

11. Harper, B., & Arms, S. (2005). *Gentle Birth Choices* (New Edition of Gentle Birth Choices Boxed Set ed.). Healing Arts Press.Pg. 79

12. MacDorman, M. F., & Declercq, E. (2018). Trends and state variations in out⊠of⊠hospital births in the United States,

2004–2017. Birth, 46(2), 279–288. https://doi.org/10.1111/birt.12411

13. Wolf, J. H. (2003). Low Breastfeeding Rates and Public Health in the United States. American Journal of Public Health, 93(12), 2000–2010. https://doi.org/10.2105/ajph.93.12.2000

14. Marylynn Salmon, "The Cultural Significance of Breastfeeding and Infant Care in Early Modern England and America," *Journal of Social History* 28 (Winter 1994): 247–269.

15. *2020 Breastfeeding Report Card.* (2020, September 17). Centers for Disease Control and Prevention. https://www.cdc.gov/breastfeeding/data/reportcard.htm

16. *USBC: Healthy People 2020: Breastfeeding Objectives.* (n.d.). US Breastfeeding Committee. Retrieved March 10, 2021, from http://www.usbreastfeeding.org/p/cm/ld/fid=221

17. Bracken-Hull, Jen (2013) "Feminism, Breastfeeding, and Society," AWE (A Woman's Experience): Vol. 1, https://scholarsarchive.byu.edu/awe/vol1/iss1/8

18. Wolf, J. B. (2010). *Is Breast Best?: Taking on the Breastfeeding Experts and the New High Stakes of Motherhood* (Biopolitics, 4). NYU Press.

CHAPTER FOUR

1. *Frequently Asked Questions—Break Time for Nursing Mothers* | U.S. Department of Labor. (n.d.). US Department of Labor. Retrieved November 7, 2020, from https://www.dol.gov/agencies/whd/nursing-mothers/faq

2. Charen, M., Hasson, M. R., Walker, A. T., Anderson, R. T., Anderson, R. T., Bachiochi, E., Charen, M., Charen, M., & Charen, M. (2018, June 28). *The Price of Feminism.* Ethics

& Public Policy Center. https://eppc.org/publications/the-price-of-feminism/

3. *Worldwide Strengths Statistics by Gender, Generation, and Country.* (2019, December 29). Chris Heinze Co. https://www.chrisheinz.com/blog/worldwide-strengths-statistics-by-gender-generation-and-country

CHAPTER FIVE

1. Taylor, J. B. (2008, April 1). *Breastfeeding is normal, formula is inferior, and birth makes the difference.* Rome New Tribune. https://www.northwestgeorgianews.com/jeannie-babb-taylor-breastfeeding-is-normal-formula-is-inferior-and-birth-makes-the-differenc-local/article_6c831346-b239-507b-b39b-c549fd5d52bb.html

2. World Health Organization. (2020, October 28). *Women's health.* https://www.who.int/health-topics/women-s-health/

3. Cavazos-Rehg, P. A., Krauss, M. J., Spitznagel, E. L., Bommarito, K., Madden, T., Olsen, M. A., Subramaniam, H., Peipert, J. F., & Bierut, L. J. (2014). Maternal Age and Risk of Labor and Delivery Complications. Maternal and Child Health Journal, 19(6), 1202–1211. https://doi.org/10.1007/s10995-014-1624-7

4. Lothian, J. A. (2005). The Birth of a Breastfeeding Baby and Mother. *Journal of Perinatal Education*, 14(1), 42–45. https://doi.org/10.1624/105812405x23667

5. Kapp, N., & Curtis, K. M. (2010). Combined oral contraceptive use among breastfeeding women: a systematic review. *Contraception,* 82(1), 10–16. https://doi.org/10.1016/j.contraception.2010.02.001

6. NHS website. (2018, October 3). *Natural family planning (fertility awareness)*. Nhs.Uk. https://www.nhs.uk/conditions/contraception/natural-family-planning/

7. M. (2011, August 2). *How do I become an abortion doula?* Radical Doula. https://radicaldoula.com/2011/08/02/how-do-i-become-an-abortion-doula/

8. Gim, E. (2021, February 15). *Led by Black Midwives, This Abortion Clinic and Birth Center Is Reimagining Health Care in the South.* Rewire News Group. https://rewirenewsgroup.com/article/2020/10/19/led-by-black-midwives-this-abortion-clinic-and-birth-center-is-reimagining-health-care-in-the-south/

9. *Buffalo Women Services: Obstetrics Gynecology: Buffalo, NY.* (n.d.). Buffalo Women Services. Retrieved November 11, 2020, from https://www.buffalowomenservices.com/

10. Phillips, Susan. (1995). The social context of women's health: Goals and objectives for medical education. CMAJ: Canadian Medical Association journal = journal de l'Association medicale canadienne. 152. 507-11.

11. World Health Organization. (2016). *Prevalence of female genital mutilation.* https://www.who.int/teams/sexual-and-reproductive-health-and-research/areas-of-work/female-genital-mutilation/prevalence-of-female-genital-mutilation

12. Edge, R. S., & Groves, J. R. (2017). *Ethics of Health Care: A Guide for Clinical Practice* (4th ed.). Cengage Learning.

13. Daniels, K., & Abma, J. (2018, December). *Products - Data Briefs - Number 327 -* December 2018. CDC. https://www.cdc.gov/nchs/products/databriefs/db327.htm

14. Burch, B. (2017, December 12). *A Medical Update on FABMS: For Physicians*. FACTS. https://www.factsaboutfertility. org/a-medical-update-on-fabms-for-physicians/

CHAPTER SIX

1. "That's Not My FACE" article in the UMD student newspaper *UMD Statesman*, accessed in 2005 (article is no longer found on the university's website).

2. Freeman, L. (2009). *Physiologic pathways of mind-body communication*. In L Freeman, ed., Mosby's Complementary and Alternative Medicine: A Research-Based Approach, 3rd ed., pp. 1–29. St. Louis: Mosby Elsevier.

3. https://www.uofmhealth.org/health-library/ mente#:~:text=If%20you're%20sick%20but,boost%20your%20 body's%20healing%20power.&text=Negative%20thoughts%20 and%20emotions%20can,that%20help%20your%20body%20 heal. Patrice Burgess, MD, FAAFP - Family Medicine & Kathleen Romito, MD - Family Medicine & Adam Husney, MD - Family Medicine & Christine R. Maldonado, PhD - Behavioral Health.

4. van der Kolk, B. A. <u>The Body Keeps the Score: Brain, Mind, and Body in the Healing of Trauma</u> (2014).

5. Ferguson, C. (2015, January 21). *How Your Mind Works and Why It's Important to Know –*. Caroline Ferguson, Mindset Trainer. https://carolineferguson.com/how-your-mind-works/#:%7E:text=Your%20brain%20has%20all%20 the,processing%20resources%20of%20your%20brain.

6. *11 Facts About Body Image*. (n.d.). DoSomething.Org. Retrieved July 7, 2020, from https://www.dosomething.org/us/

facts/11-facts-about-body-image#:%7E:text=Approximately%20
91%25%20of%20women%20are,to%20be%20a%20certain%20
weight.

7. Collins, M. E. (1991). *Body figure perceptions and preferences among preadolescent children.* International Journal of Eating Disorders, 10(2), 199–208. https://doi.org/10.1002/1098-108X(199103)10:2<199::AID-EAT2260100209>3.0.CO;2-D

8. National Organization for Women. (2014, November 29). Get The Facts. https://now.org/now-foundation/love-your-body/love-your-body-whats-it-all-about/get-the-facts/#:%7E:text=46%25%20of%209%2D11%20year,looks%20after%20reading%20women's%20magazines.

9. van der Kolk, B. A. The Body Keeps the Score: Brain, Mind, and Body in the Healing of Trauma (2014). Pg. 81.

CHAPTER SEVEN

1. Miller, A. E. J., MacDougall, J. D., Tarnopolsky, M. A., & Sale, D. G. (1993). Gender differences in strength and muscle fiber characteristics. *European Journal of Applied Physiology and Occupational Physiology*, 66(3), 254–262. https://doi.org/10.1007/bf00235103

2. Nast, C. (2016, January 13). *Caitlyn Jenner Glamour Women of the Year 2015 Award Acceptance Speech.* Glamour. https://www.glamour.com/story/caitlyn-jenner-speech

3. Beauvoir, S. (2015). *The Second Sex (Vintage Feminism Short Edition)* (2015-03-20) [Paperback]. Vintage Classics.

4. Regalado, A. (2020, June 19). *More than 26 million people have taken an at-home ancestry test.* MIT Technology Review. https://

www.technologyreview.com/2019/02/11/103446/more-than-26-million-people-have-taken-an-at-home-ancestry-test/

CHAPTER EIGHT

1. Fulwiler, J., & Gaffigan, J. (2020). *Your Blue Flame: Drop the Guilt and Do What Makes You Come Alive.* (1st ed.). Zondervan.

2. Ibid.

3. nmcnews24. (2019, August 2). *Australian senator breastfeeds baby in parliament.* http://nmcnews24.com/2019/08/02/the-three-month-old-previously-made-history-in-may-after-she-became-the-first-baby-to-be-breastfed-in-australias/

4. Gale, R. (2019, December 13). *The Other Backroom: Breast-Feeding on the Hill.* Roll Call. https://www.rollcall.com/2014/02/02/the-other-backroom-breast-feeding-on-the-hill/

5. Aldridge, B. (2021, January 4). *No more 'he' or 'she'. House approves gender-neutral terms in its official language.* McClatchty DC Bureau. https://www.mcclatchydc.com/news/politics-government/article248264460.html

6. Ibid.

7. Friedman, D. (2017, July 14). *Perk Up: Facebook and Apple Now Pay for Women to Freeze Eggs.* NBC News. https://www.nbcnews.com/news/us-news/perk-facebook-apple-now-pay-women-freeze-eggs-n225011